CYSTIC FIBROSIS

HUMAN HORIZONS SERIES

CYSTIC FIBROSIS

A Guide for Parents and Sufferers

Percy Bray

with a Foreword by
Sir Eric Stroud, FRCP
Professor Emeritus, King's College, London
and Hon Medical Director Children Nationwide
Medical Research Fund

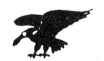

A CONDOR BOOK
SOUVENIR PRESS (E & A) LTD

ISBN 0 285 65077 7 hardback
ISBN 0 285 65076 9 paperback

Photoset by Rowland Phototypesetting Ltd,
Bury St Edmunds, Suffolk
Printed in Great Britain by
WBC Bristol and Maesteg

FOREWORD

Percy Bray was an outstanding paediatrician. His clinical skills and breadth of knowledge were equalled by an ability to teach and motivate those who worked under his careful and kind guidance. For many of us the decision to follow a career in paediatrics was in large part due to the admiration which, as students, we held for him. We benefited from his erudition and also from the compassion and loving responsibility which he felt towards his child patients and their families. His ability to explain complex disease states and to be sensitive to our own and patients' anxieties made him the great teacher of whom we were all proud. Indeed many of us regretted that he did not widen, by writing, the audience for his talents.

This present publication illustrates much of Percy's quality and it is appropriate that this is done through a book, the objective of which is to explain fully to children, adults and their families a disease which was Percy Bray's major interest.

The recent advances in the area of genetic diseases have added to the hope for the future in Cystic Fibrosis in terms of prevention and cure. In addition, advances in treatment have enabled the majority of Cystic Fibrosis children to grow up into active adult life.

Percy Bray has used his great gift for communication to explain the patho-physiology of the genetic mechanisms, presentation and clinical care of Cystic Fibrosis.

He analyses very cleverly the emotional responses of patients and parents; in particular he describes in a factual and kindly way the anxieties which occur at the time of adolescence.

Finally he describes with typical optimism his view of the future.

Percy's death was unexpected and a great sadness to his family and friends. This book in a few clinical matters will become out of date. As a careful, compassionate and extremely helpful aid to all those who suffer from or are otherwise concerned with Cystic Fibrosis, it will always be a symbol of the dedication shown by Percy Bray in his lifetime.

C. Eric Stroud

PUBLISHER'S NOTE

Sadly, Professor Bray died shortly after completing the main text of this book and before he had had time to write any acknowledgements to the many people who had helped him in its preparation. Rather than risk offending anyone who may have provided help, and whose name we do not have, we thought it best, with the agreement of the author's family, to offer here a general statement of appreciation and thanks to those who have made a contribution to the book, whether by providing advice, information and illustrations, or by giving permission for their material or illustrations to be reproduced.

We should, however, like to make special mention of two people whose help has been invaluable, both while the book was being written and in preparing it for the printers. Mrs Barbara Bentley, Director of the Cystic Fibrosis Research Trust, has been unstinting in her help and advice and has allowed material owned by the Trust to be used in the book. She also very kindly prepared the Glossary and Bibliography, giving up her holiday to meet the printers' deadline. Mrs Marilyn Morgan typed the whole manuscript and was closely involved in the research and writing. She has been enormously helpful in tying up loose ends to complete the book as the author would have wished.

To both these kind people, to Professor Eric Stroud for agreeing to write a Foreword to the book, and to all those whose names we cannot trace but who contributed in many different ways, we offer our sincere thanks.

CONTENTS

INTRODUCTION

Being told, however kindly, that your baby has been born with an incurable inherited disease is inevitably a tragic and traumatic experience—especially so when the condition is relatively rare and unfamiliar to most people.

Cystic Fibrosis is a long-term, life-threatening disease affecting the lungs and digestive system, and at present there is no cure. But over the years increasingly effective techniques of management and treatment have been developed, involving both parents and patients, which have changed the likelihood of Cystic Fibrosis babies from dying in early childhood to a 75 per cent chance of reaching adulthood. These positive developments give me great confidence and make me feel hopeful about the future. This conviction of hope is one thing that has enabled me to stay so long in the field of Cystic Fibrosis.

My real knowledge of what was then a recently recognised disease began in 1946, at Great Ormond Street Hospital, where I was privileged to work for several years with some of the pioneers in Cystic Fibrosis research, Dr A. P. Norman, Dr David Lawson and Dr Martin Bodian. Over the next forty years, during which my involvement with Cystic Fibrosis continued, I came to appreciate and admire the courage, gumption and loving, dedicated support that parents can summon up in the face of apparent disaster. The ways in which Cystic Fibrosis children and adolescents have coped with their situation, minimising suffering and disability, but determined to develop their potential assets, compelled my respect and admiration.

This book sets out first to provide parents with essential information about Cystic Fibrosis: what it is, how it is inherited, what goes wrong in the various organs and tissues of the body, what the symptoms are and how the disease is diagnosed. The first two chapters deal necessarily with medical and scientific aspects. I make no apology for this, as I believe that parents (and patients in due course) have a right to be told the main facts of our present knowledge of the disease, expressed in non-technical language. You will in any case read or hear such words as 'pancreatic pathology', 'sweat electrolytes', 'meconium ileus' and so on. The better you know the essential scientific facts, the better equipped you will be to cope with the requirements of the 'whole child' treatment, which success-ful management of a long-term life-threatening illness requires.

The major part of the book deals with management. I shall describe first what I consider to be the general prin-ciples and the overall strategy, then the individualised and comprehensive ongoing programme of 'shared care'. The practical aspects of this, which involve parents, patients and what I have called the 'caregivers' network', will be discussed in detail, and I shall stress the importance of promoting healthy activities, with special reference to the best possible functioning of the vital respiratory tract. The psychosocial aspects of Cystic Fibrosis will be considered, using some case histories from my own clinical experience. Education requires a section to itself, as do adolescents and adults with Cystic Fibrosis, since their treatment is becoming increasingly important.

No book about Cystic Fibrosis, for families and patients of all ages, would be complete without an account of the Cystic Fibrosis Research Trust, with its headquarters at Bromley and local branches throughout the United Kingdom.

Finally, I shall dare to dip into the future: Hopefully to glimpse the promise just visible on this particular Human Horizon.

1   WHAT IS CYSTIC FIBROSIS?

James was the first child of a young couple, Alan and Barbara, who were both healthy, active and intelligent. They were delighted with their fine baby son and full of great hopes for his future. But by the time he was one year old, it had become clear that all was not well with his health. He had suffered a series of what were taken to be 'coughs and colds', and now had a persistent cough, especially in the morning, occasionally accompanied by slight wheezing and sometimes vomiting. In spite of a good appetite and a fully adequate diet, his weight gain was not up to normal; also, Barbara noticed that his bowel motions were frequent, bulky and greasy-looking, with a peculiarly unpleasant smell.

The doctor at the clinic thought James's case should be investigated further, so the family doctor looked him over and then referred him to the consultant paediatrician at the district hospital. The specialist examined him and told his parents he was arranging further special tests and would see them all the following week.

Most of the tests, including X-rays, were done immediately; one, however, which rather puzzled the family, was carried out a few days later. They were told this was a 'Sweat Test'. On their next visit the paediatrician told them that James was suffering from CYSTIC FIBROSIS. They knew virtually nothing about this, apart from some posters Alan had seen, a paragraph or two in the newspaper and a few the odd mention on television. The paediatrician arranged to see them again the next day for a further discussion.

Later that afternoon they took James home. Alan drove, Barbara sitting quietly at his side, saying nothing. James, in his safety seat in the back, was tired and sleepy. After a while he started a coughing bout and was sick and crying. Alan stopped. Barbara went to the back seat, took James in her arms, cleaned him up, and nursed him as she had when he was first born; now, however, she was weeping silently. James went back to sleep.

When they arrived home, they saw to James, who fed well and went to sleep as usual on being put to bed. His parents went downstairs and sat silently for a time.

'I can hardly believe it,' said Barbara. 'What is it? What does it mean? What can we do? I feel so helpless.'

'I don't really know,' said Alan. 'They will tell us all about it tomorrow, I expect. I think I'll give George a ring (a business friend). I think they had a case in his family.' He returned some minutes later. 'He says it's a type of hereditary condition that affects the stomach and the lungs, and most children get pneumonia and don't live very long.'

The only family member who slept at all well that night was James. Next morning he ate his breakfast of cereal, rusks and milk without coughing or vomiting, but quickly filled his nappy. Something prompted Barbara to save it and take it with her to the hospital; it was just the sort of motion she had noticed previously—very large, greasy and quite offensive.

They arrived early for their appointment, but were taken immediately to the paediatrician's office next to which was a playroom. James was placed in the charge of the 'play-lady', and Barbara could see him all the time through the large glass door; more important, he could see her. The 'play-lady' introduced him to a little girl aged about four, and James (who could walk quite well—he was now 15 months) went and picked up a doll from the floor and presented it to her.

With the paediatrician was another doctor who was introduced as the Consultant in charge of the Regional Unit for Cystic Fibrosis at the University Hospital, ten miles away.

Since the previous day Barbara and Alan felt that their world had fallen apart; Barbara, especially, experienced feelings of intense grief, anxiety, self-doubt and guilt; Alan too felt shocked, worried, and resentful against the fate that had brought this disaster on them.

James was now coughing and crying, beating on the glass door. Barbara quickly dried her tears, feeling a tremendous upsurge of love and protectiveness towards him as she went quickly and took him from the play-lady. The doctors placed them in an armchair and left them alone together, taking Alan into a side-room. The Regional Consultant told Alan that they would like James to come into the Cystic Fibrosis Unit at the University Hospital for a short time, to enable a total evaluation of his condition to be made, with special and detailed attention to the lungs; they would then work out with Alan and Barbara a programme of ongoing comprehensive care, in which the parents would play an important part.

'Of course,' he said to Alan, 'you are both welcome to come and be with James as much as you like, and your wife can stay at night if she likes. We are going to meet often, and it will be an important part of my job to give you full information about Cystic Fibrosis in general, and James's case in particular. At the same time you will receive practical instruction in physiotherapy and dietary management, and will practise the various procedures under supervision.'

Barbara had now rejoined them. 'First of all,' she said, 'I'd like to know exactly what Cystic Fibrosis is. What causes it? Could it have been prevented? What symptoms can we expect to see? Is there a cure?'

They returned to the main office and, while James went back to the playroom, the parents and doctors sat round and heard the Consultant outline the programme which he hoped they would approve. He gave them some notes to study at home and began the first of many 'tutorials' with some general information about Cystic Fibrosis. The notes included:

1 The type of inheritance (Genetics).
2 What goes wrong in various parts of the body (Pathology).

3   What the different symptoms are (Clinical).
4   How the disease is diagnosed.

The doctors told them how the care of James's case would be shared between the Cystic Fibrosis centre and the district hospital and home services. So James was admitted to the unit and began his long association with the team there. Alan and Barbara heard how the outlook for Cystic Fibrosis children had improved over the last two decades, and for the first time they felt some reassurance and hope for the future.

*   *   *

Cystic Fibrosis is the name used today to denote the commonest inherited disorder affecting children in Europe and North America. Recognition is based upon an idea and concept formulated in 1938 by Dr Dorothy Andersen, who brought together the case histories of numerous babies and young children who had suffered a mysterious illness-complex with varied symptoms, including general failure to thrive, digestional problems and progressive chest disease, leading in most cases to early death. She believed that there was a common underlying defect, and when she came to examine the pancreas gland in all these cases, she found abnormal appearances resembling cysts, together with overgrowth of tissue fibres around the groups of cells which secrete the important digestive juices. These findings gave rise to the original name 'Fibrocystic Disease of the Pancreas'. Further studies showed that the digestive juices were unusually viscous and 'sticky', tending to block the ducts carrying them from the pancreas to the small intestine, where they would play a major part in the digestive process.

It also became recognised that it was repeated chest infections and bronchitis which were responsible for serious ill health and early death. Here, too, the mucous secretions in the bronchial tubes were thick, sticky and abnormally viscid. What was intended by nature to be thin and lubricating became unduly thick and blocking in this disease—hence the alternative designation still used on the Continent: 'Mucoviscidosis' (Mukoviscidösc).

Delving into the medical history in Europe, we find that as far back as 1905, Professor Landsteiner in Vienna had described similar cases in newborn babies, as had Professor Fanconi (Virchow's Archives) in 1920. Mediaeval German folklore includes a saying concerning young infants: 'Sad for the babe, whose face when kissed, salty tastes: it is bewitched, and soon must die.' This is another facet of Cystic Fibrosis—the markedly increased concentration of sodium chloride in the sweat, present from birth, which forms the basis for the most commonly used diagnostic test for the disease, the Sweat Test. Salt is water retentive, and in hot countries where humidity is high, sufferers are liable to 'heat exhaustion' due to the excessive salt loss in their sweat and the resulting dehydration.

The racial incidence of Cystic Fibrosis is interesting: the disease is most common in 'Caucasian' peoples—that is fair-skinned races—but is also found in peoples of North Africa and Western Asia. In the United Kingdom the incidence is about 1:2,500 live births. A few cases are known in Afro-Caribbeans and the author has encountered four fully diagnosed cases in Chinese and Malay children. At the Budapest Cystic Fibrosis conference in 1986, Professor Yamashura presented data from 81 Japanese patients.

How Cystic Fibrosis is Inherited

Cystic Fibrosis is the commonest genetically determined disease in the United Kingdom, so it is important for parents, and in due course the patients, to understand how it is inherited.

Genes may be regarded as the units of inheritance. They are carried in, and transported by, structures known as chromosomes, found in the nucleus of every human cell. The body cells (but not the sperms or eggs) contain two identical or nearly identical sets of chromosomes—one derived from the egg, the other from the sperm—and during the formation of the reproductive cells the number of chromosomes in them is reduced to half. The genes, composed of complex molecules (DNA) are arranged on the chromosomes in linear fashion, like beads, and occupy definite positions (loci) which can sometimes be ascertained and mapped. They carry a code or blue-print to the offspring for the production of a particular protein or enzyme. The genes in body cells exist in pairs, one gene from each parent. If the genes are similar the condition is termed 'homozygous'; if dissimilar, it is 'heterozygous', for that gene. Some genes are termed 'dominant'—that is to say, when a pair is heterozygous it will be the dominant gene whose products will be shown in the child. Other genes (the Cystic Fibrosis gene is one) only have their say, so to speak, if neither member of the gene pair is dominant —termed 'recessive'. Therefore, Cystic Fibrosis is inherited as 'autosomal' (body cells) 'recessive'.

It follows from this that the Cystic Fibrosis child is homozygous for the Cystic Fibrosis gene; and that both parents are heterozygotes: healthy 'carriers' of the gene.

So far we have encountered about half a dozen words with which the average parent will never have had any need to be familiar. This, together with the natural anxiety, apprehension and depression associated with the discovery that one's child has been born with an incurable hereditary disease, which could happen again in the next pregnancy, makes many people switch off as further genetic jargon overwhelms them.

Nevertheless, I think it is important that families in which Cystic Fibrosis has appeared should gain an understanding of the principles of human inheritance and the mechanisms of genetics. They have a right to this, so that the various questions which inevitably crop up at some time or another, among parents, children, prospective partners and other relatives, can be fairly considered and genetic counselling fully appreciated.

My aim here is therefore to explain the inheritance of Cystic Fibrosis in such a way as to make the basic principles understandable by everyone. Then, in Chapter Five, after you have read the chapters on symptoms and treatment of

Cystic Fibrosis, a more detailed exposition of human genetics is provided, together with questions and answers from a number of actual case histories. By that time I think you will know enough about Cystic Fibrosis, and will have discussed it with others, to want to know the answers to questions like those below:

What is the chance I could be a carrier?
—My mother is CF.
—My sister (or brother) is CF.
—My sister (or brother) has a Cystic Fibrosis baby.
—My mother (or father) was married before, and my half-sister (or brother) has Cystic Fibrosis.
—There is no history of Cystic Fibrosis in my family.
—When will an accurate diagnostic test for Cystic Fibrosis be available?

What is the chance we could have a Cystic Fibrosis baby?
—There is no Cystic Fibrosis in the history of either of our families.
—My sister (or brother) has Cystic Fibrosis; my partner has no family history of the disease.
—My sister (or brother) has a Cystic Fibrosis baby; my partner has no such history.
—My mother (or father) had a Cystic Fibrosis child by her previous marriage; my partner has no history of Cystic Fibrosis in the family.
—My mother is CF: I am healthy and my partner also, and there is no family history there.
—My partner and I are first cousins; there is no family history of Cystic Fibrosis.
—We already have one child with Cystic Fibrosis (recently diagnosed).
—What is the present situation regarding accurate prenatal diagnosis in early pregnancy?

Saying that Cystic Fibrosis is a genetic disease means that it is passed from generation to generation in families. It is important for you to understand that people can carry an inherited disease and not display any of the symptoms. There may not be any history of Cystic Fibrosis in their family. This is quite usual in Cystic Fibrosis and other genetic diseases where two doses of the abnormal gene are necessary before the condition shows itself as an illness with the typical symptoms. This is a RECESSIVE DISEASE. It means that both mother and father of a Cystic Fibrosis child will carry one Cystic Fibrosis gene in each and every body cell but also one normal gene, which is what we mean when we say they are HETEROZYGOUS for the gene. In Cystic Fibrosis carriers, however, the normal gene in the parents is DOMINANT—that is to say, the normal gene in the parents takes over and does what the Cystic Fibrosis gene should have done, so that no ill-effects occur. The one Cystic Fibrosis gene does not exert any effects: it is RECESSIVE. But all sufferers from Cystic Fibrosis carry two Cystic Fibrosis genes in every cell, one inherited from their mother and the second from the father. We say they are HOMOZYGOUS for the Cystic Fibrosis gene which therefore has no dominant normal gene to countermand it; the abnormal gene effect is then produced, leading to the symptoms of Cystic Fibrosis.

In the same way, for the mother and father each to have one Cystic Fibrosis gene, it must have been inherited from one of their parents, who were also single Cystic Fibrosis gene carriers and will have shown no symptoms of the disease.

Thus the Cystic Fibrosis gene is passed from generation to generation without symptoms being apparent.

The Cystic Fibrosis gene is indeed very common. Geneticists estimate that two and a half million men and women in Britain are healthy carriers—that is, about one in twenty-five people carry a single Cystic Fibrosis gene. Generally these people would never know unless they mated with another gene carrier (the statistical chance of this is one in 625, or 624 to one against) and produced an affected child. The present situation regarding the availability of a reliable diagnostic test for Cystic Fibrosis heterozygote gene carriers is described in more detail later; I would only say here that those people who know now that they must be carriers will almost certainly have received some genetic counselling. At first, the psychological and perhaps social consequences of knowing one is a carrier are likely to affect one's full understanding of the implications of the news, and this important aspect of the matter is also dealt with in Chapters Three and Six. Figure 1 illustrates the chances for the offspring of two Cystic Fibrosis carriers.

The chances of two unrelated carriers (not first cousins) meeting and having children are:

$$1/25 \times 1/25 = 1 \text{ in } 625$$

There is a one in four chance that both parents could pass this single Cystic Fibrosis gene to one of their children, who would then be homozygous for the recessive gene and would suffer from the disease Cystic Fibrosis. There is also a one in four chance that each parent could contribute his or her normal gene to a child, who would then be quite normal genetically, and of course completely free from Cystic Fibrosis.

Another possibility is that one Cystic Fibrosis gene and one normal gene could pass to each of two children, who would then be heterozygote Cystic Fibrosis carriers but themselves healthy and normal.

To sum up: of the one in 625 couples who are both Cystic Fibrosis carriers, there is a one in four chance of producing a Cystic Fibrosis child, a two in four chance of a child being a carrier and a one in four chance of having a child free from the Cystic Fibrosis gene altogether.

It is estimated that at present about 650,000 births occur annually. The statistical chance of having a Cystic Fibrosis baby is:

$$1/25 \times 1/25 \times 1/4 = 1/2,500$$

This would give $650,000 \div 2,500 = 260$ Cystic Fibrosis births born each year, a figure which agrees with the estimate of Professor John Dodge who is collecting a computer database for Cystic Fibrosis throughout the United Kingdom.

It is important for you to realise that the various chances, of being a Cystic Fibrosis carrier, or having a Cystic Fibrosis

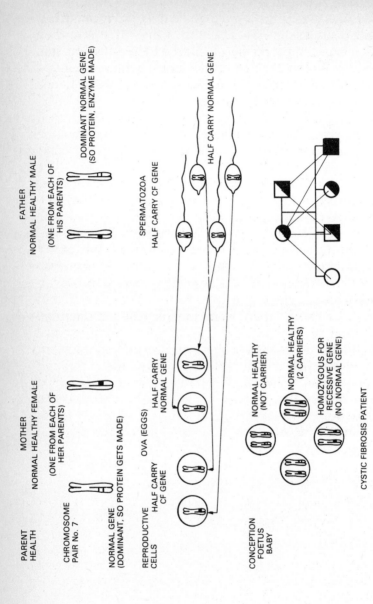

Figure 1. Genetic sequence leading to a Cystic Fibrosis baby. We do not *yet* know what protein is normally made on instruction from the normal gene at Cystic Fibrosis Locus on Chromosome 7.

baby, given as one in two, two in three, or one in four, are theoretical statistical risks only, and it does not mean that if a couple has a Cystic Fibrosis child for their firstborn, they can then expect the next three children to be either carriers or completely free of the Cystic Fibrosis gene. For such a couple, who are definite Cystic Fibrosis carriers, the chance of having a Cystic Fibrosis baby are one in four for each and every pregnancy.

Having read this introduction to genetics, there will be many questions which you will want to put to your doctor in the Cystic Fibrosis clinic. Some will be urgent—for example, your brother's wife may just have had a baby which turns out to have Cystic Fibrosis, and you believe that you may be pregnant. You will be anxious to know whether you might have a Cystic Fibrosis baby and what you should do. Other questions will be more scientific. Many people want to know what the Cystic Fibrosis gene is, what it is made of, where it is, how it makes a child ill, what can be done about it. These questions have a very practical and a significant basis, apart from the request for scientific information.

I shall attempt to answer these and related enquiries in Chapter Five. What is called 'The New Genetics' is making progress by very many little steps and now and then a big step forward, advancing both our knowledge and ability to diagnose and treat Cystic Fibrosis in a radical and much more hopeful manner.

2 WHAT GOES WRONG IN CYSTIC FIBROSIS?

As I indicated in Chapter One, Cystic Fibrosis affects certain organs of the body, causing malfunction and symptoms of ill-health. In this chapter I shall look at the way the organs are affected and the resulting sensations and signs which the doctor may see (sometimes called 'clinical findings') and which may worry the parents and make the patient feel unwell.

How the Body is Affected

The Pancreas
This organ lies on the back of the abdomen, behind the stomach. Under the microscope it can be seen to be composed of groups of cells which make the digestive juices and secrete them into small channels (ducts); these join up to make the main pancreatic ducts which open into the upper part of the intestine (duodenum), together with the bile duct. In Cystic Fibrosis the pancreas organ can be seen to show blockage and dilatation of the ducts (resembling, but not actually, cysts); there is also degeneration (due to back pressure?) of the important secretory cells, and increased fibrous tissue (see Figure 2).

The Lungs
These appear generally normal at birth, apart from enlarged mucus glands. Later, the abnormally sticky, viscid mucus blocks some of the smaller air-tubes (bronchioles), sometimes completely so that the piece of lung served by that airway becomes quite airless and collapsed (atelectasis); or the mucus partially blocks the bronchial tube so that air can get into the piece of lung but not out again, so

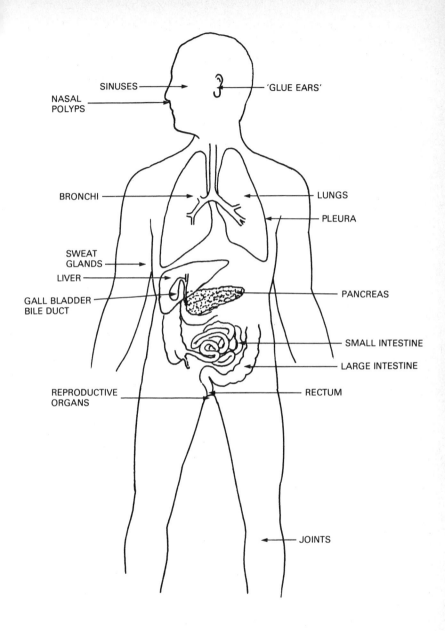

Figure 2. The parts of the body principally affected in Cystic Fibrosis.

there is air-trapping and blown-up portions of lung (emphysema) (see Figure 2).

All this leads to impaired clearance of the lungs and airways, in spite of coughing; and infection easily occurs, leading to further progressive lung damage, attacks of pneumonia and lung abscess. The sputum becomes a mixture of mucus and pus. Some unusual bacteria are found, suggesting impaired defence mechanisms in the chest. Similar changes occur in the upper respiratory tract (the nose and sinuses).

Sweat Glands

Unlike the pancreas and respiratory tract, the sweat glands in Cystic Fibrosis show no evident abnormality, even under the electron microscope. The sweat secretion is derived from the blood, where salt is present in a strength of over 100 units. Normally, during the passage of sweat from the base of the gland to the skin, most of the salt is reabsorbed so that sweat coming out from the pores on the surface contains less than 40 units (see Figure 2). Something is thought to go wrong with the reabsorption process in Cystic Fibrosis, so that the surface sweat contains 80–120 units. As already described, this renders Cystic Fibrosis patients liable to heat exhaustion, with dehydration and salt loss. The use of the sweat abnormality in diagnosing Cystic Fibrosis is described in the next chapter.

Sex Organs

In girls, the ovaries, tubes, and body of the uterus are normal for age, although the onset of menstruation is often delayed. Conception may be made difficult by distension and tenacious mucus accumulation in the cervix.

In boys, the structure and ducts which store and then transmit the spermatozoa from the testes on their circuitous journey to the exterior and the female vagina, are poorly developed and even absent in some parts, so that few or no sperms are available. Cystic Fibrosis males are therefore almost always infertile; but not impotent, and sexual intercourse can take place in the normal way.

Symptoms

These are described, first, according to the organ systems from which they arise, for example, digestive, nutritional, respiratory; secondly, according to the way Cystic Fibrosis commonly presents at different times of life, the 'Seven Ages' of Cystic Fibrosis.

Respiratory Tract

The first symptom most commonly noticed by the mother is the child's cough. At first this may be intermittent, dry and hacking in nature, worse at night or on waking. As the condition worsens the cough becomes more persistent and sounds looser. Babies and small children do not expectorate phlegm as a rule, but in Cystic Fibrosis paroxysms of coughing, resembling Whooping Cough, often occur as the disease develops; and like that infection, the paroxysms may end in vomiting. The vomit may be seen to contain phlegm, which has been swallowed after passing up from the chest to the throat. This 'sputum' is thick and sticky, with pus mixed in with the bronchial mucus. About this time, also, parents may notice the child wheezing during or following bouts of coughing, and he may become short of breath with the wheezing, especially on exertion. Attacks of chest infection occur as time goes on, with raised temperature and breathing rate, worsening cough and phlegm. The doctor examining the child with a stethoscope hears various abnormal sounds in the chest; a chest X-ray will show some, or many, small or large shadows, and laboratory tests on the phlegm indicate infection, not with the classic pneumococcus bacteria, but various bacteria with strange names such as staphylococcus, pseudomonas, klebsiella and other exotic strains, which as a rule only rarely cause lung infections. As the chest trouble gets worse, the child loses appetite and weight.

When describing the chest symptoms in Cystic Fibrosis, it is easy to forget that the respiratory tract begins at the tip of the nose and extends through the nostrils and the nasal cavities, into which open those cavernous extensions into the facial bones and base of the skull, known as the paranasal sinuses. All those spaces are lined with warm, moist tissues which serve to warm and humidify the air we breathe in. There are also cleansing mechanisms in the nose, sinuses, and back of the throat, so that with proper nasal breathing the air reaches the main chest airways and lungs in the best possible condition. In Cystic Fibrosis changes occur in the upper respiratory tract resembling those described in the bronchi and lungs. The mucus-secreting glands are enlarged and the secretion is thick and viscous, not easily drained away, and tending to block the nasal passages; infection easily occurs, leading to sinusitis and chronic nasal congestion.

The gland-bearing tissues tend to develop benign 'over-growths' (lumps on stalks), producing 'nasal polyps' which further aggravate the situation. On going to bed and lying down to sleep, the child is bothered by nasal discharge from the back of the nose and throat running down and irritating the larynx, so that violent bouts of night coughing become a troublesome symptom. Nasal polyps are generally rare in children, and their occurrence should point to the need for diagnostic tests for Cystic Fibrosis. Nasal polyps are also a feature of allergic conditions such as Hay Fever and Asthma, and evidence of respiratory allergy is often found in Cystic Fibrosis patients with nasal polyps. This 'bronchial lability' is important in the diagnosis and treatment of Cystic Fibrosis.

Digestion
One of the features of this disease is that the onset of the different symptoms and their degree of severity vary from patient to patient.

The old saying that Cystic Fibrosis is characterised by 'failure to thrive in spite of a large appetite' is not true in all cases, although it is true that in the early years, before respiratory infections have set in, the height and weight of Cystic Fibrosis children is below average. Part of the reason for this can be found in the child's bowel motions. Three to five times a day, the child will pass stools which are loose, bulky, pale, greasy-looking or even oily, perhaps with some undigested food, and with a characteristic and unpleasant odour. The motions may be difficult to remove from the napkin or to flush down the pan. A few patients have sufficient pancreatic enzyme production during the first year or so to produce normal stools, but as a rule this declines steadily over the next few years.

The child's abdomen appears somewhat distended, at first only occasionally, but later more prominently and permanently, contrasting with the relatively skinny limbs and unusually flat buttocks. Vomiting is not especially common, but may occur with coughing. There may be attacks of abdominal pain, particularly in older children, and they may sometimes be quite severe and require special treatment.

Laboratory tests will indicate some degree of pancreatic enzyme deficiency, from slight to severe, occasionally complete absence. Rarely in adolescent patients, but more commonly in adults, attacks of pancreatitis may occur and are occasionally followed by development of stones (calculi) in the organ.

The liver is affected by the sticky viscid bile plugging the ducts, together with the formation of excess fibrous tissue and deposition of fat. This very rarely causes trouble until adult life, although the liver can be felt to be enlarged to some degree in about a third of older children. The severe changes and complications seen, for example, in alcoholic liver cirrhosis, are very rarely seen in Cystic Fibrosis; a recent survey showed that not more than five per cent of adult cases showed symptoms of this type. Prolapse of the lower bowel (rectal prolapse) is a common and, for the toddler and his parents, an alarming symptom in Cystic Fibrosis, and may be the first sign of the disorder. Fortunately, it should lead to early diagnosis and treatment, and the prolapse itself can be corrected without surgery.

The 'Seven Ages' of Cystic Fibrosis
Owing to the considerable variation in onset, severity and rate of progression of the different symptom complexes,

some experts have postulated several types of Cystic Fibrosis. There is, however, a general age period when certain features are more prominent, together with some less well known features which are nevertheless important to patient and family and which may present as the first indication of Cystic Fibrosis and serve as pointers to diagnosis and management.

1 The Newborn

Pregnancy usually proceeds normally: premature birth is no more than usual, but Cystic Fibrosis babies are on average 'Low Birth Weight'. Between ten and 15 per cent, however, are born with intestinal obstruction, known as 'meconium ileus': meconium is the name given to the greenish-black, sticky, semi-liquid bowel movements of the newborn over the first few days of life. (The word 'meconium' is derived from the Ancient Greek word for the opium poppy, and physicians at the time thought meconium was the poppy juice which kept the infant asleep in the womb until the time came to be born, when it was discharged.) Those Cystic Fibrosis infants afflicted with meconium ileus pass no bowel motions, the abdomen is grossly distended and vomiting soon sets in. The cause of the trouble is that the meconium in the intestine is abnormally viscous, sticky and dry (like plasticine) and blocks up the bowel passage. Meconium ileus obstruction is an emergency, necessitating transfer to a paediatric unit with appropriate surgical facilities. An operation is not always required and about a half of the cases can be treated successfully by special enemas.

One might think that with Cystic Fibrosis manifesting itself so early, and in such a potentially very serious way, the outlook for the affected child will be bad. In fact, this is not so: those patients who survive the immediate crisis (and the vast majority do survive) are known to have a slightly better outlook than average. This we will discuss further when considering the advantages of early diagnosis of Cystic Fibrosis.

2 *Early Infancy*

This is the period during which the classic symptoms described make their appearance—especially the disappointing weight gain, the harsh cough, noisy breathing and signs of bronchitis; the abnormal bowel motions (which have been present from the newborn period) are now noticed and prompt the organisation of various diagnostic tests. About 65 per cent of cases are diagnosed during this time.

3 *Later Infancy*

Up to this time, the 'mewing and puking in the nurse's arms' have not been much in evidence: Cystic Fibrosis babies are usually lively and happy, but now vomiting becomes a symptom, often with coughing on waking in the morning, and perceptive parents may notice pus in sputum with the vomited material. Cases of heat exhaustion during heat waves or feverish illnesses have been recorded.

4 *Pre-School*

Most cases of Cystic Fibrosis will have been recognised and treated by the age of four, but in those children who have not been diagnosed, or where treatment has been inadequate, the picture of 'global malnutrition' becomes evident. There is failure to gain weight, short stature, frequent loose, bulky, fatty motions; and a serious situation develops when the chest symptoms become more marked. Many children in this group present with an alarming symptom—prolapse of the bowel, or rectal prolapse. Usually following the passage of one of the abnormal bowel motions (or a coughing bout), the lining of the lowest section of the bowel turns inside out and shows as a reddish fleshy swelling protruding through the back passage; this is very sensitive and may bleed to some extent but is not especially painful, and it can be put back by lying the patient prone or on the side and exerting gentle pressure with the lubricated fingers of the gloved hand. Surgical operation is very rarely necessary. But more than this, if the diagnosis has not yet been made, the appearance of rectal prolapse in a European child should indicate the absolute necessity for Cystic Fibrosis diagnostic tests to be carried out as soon as possible. In known Cystic Fibrosis patients, rectal prolapse is an indication for review and updating of diet, pancreatic enzyme dosage, and treatment of chest symptoms.

5   *School Age*
Cystic Fibrosis children are generally bright and happy, and though they may have a 'shining morning face', they seldom creep unwillingly to school unless upset by spasms of coughing and vomiting, or perhaps those cramp-like abdominal pains which begin to afflict some Cystic Fibrosis patients in this age group.

The pains are colicky in nature and occur in recurrent bouts, usually accompanied by forcible vomiting and severe constipation. At first, the pains are usually in the centre of the abdomen; later, they appear in the right lower portion, where a firm plastic lump can often be felt. Obviously further medical examinations and X-rays are required to establish a correct diagnosis and to exclude appendix abscess. The Cystic Fibrosis condition is termed meconium ileus equivalent, because it resembles the condition in the newborn: unusually stiff, tenacious mucoid faeces collect and obstruct the small intestine at its junction with the large bowel. There is no real connection between the two conditions, however.

Having established the diagnosis and excluding conditions such as 'intussusception' (a sort of telescoping of the intestine in the same region, also not uncommon in Cystic Fibrosis), treatment is by special enemas (gastrografin) together with intravenous fluid drips: operation is very rarely required. Follow-up care includes review of diet, adjustment of the dose of pancreatic enzymes, and sometimes regular or intermittent doses of mineral oil given at bedtime.

6   *Adolescence* and 7   *Adulthood*
The increasing number of patients living to adolescence and adulthood (80 per cent overall reaching 13 years of age

and 60 per cent 20 years—more in some centres) is a cause for rejoicing and renewed hope among Cystic Fibrosis patients, their families, the profession involved and the Cystic Fibrosis Research Trust; but it also poses some new problems, especially in the psychosocial field. These merit separate attention, which is provided in Chapter Seven. Here, our concern is the clinical problems common in this age group, nearly all of whom were diagnosed in infancy or childhood; a very few, however, present for the first time with one or more of the following:

a) Chronic bronchitis, with attacks of pneumonia. Chest X-ray, sputum cultures and the sweat test are all diagnostic. Some patients in this category have reasonable pancreatic function. The author has seen a woman of 45 recently diagnosed, who fits into this sub-group.

b) Chronic Sinusitis, with polyposis and recurrent bronchitis. Known cases of Cystic Fibrosis may show these symptoms during adolescence and adulthood, also such additional disorders as:

c) Diabetes mellitus.

d) Signs of liver disease and pancreatitis.

e) The 'meconium ileus equivalent'.

f) Poor growth and poor or abnormal development.

g) Reduced fertility.

Any one or more of these physical troubles will become intertwined with the normal psychosocial adolescent problems, added to those associated with chronic disease.

3   DIAGNOSIS

The diagnosis of Cystic Fibrosis is an event of such importance in the life of the patient and the family that it should be based upon the best available tests as regards accuracy, precision, sensitivity and specificity that modern laboratory medicine can provide. 'Sensitivity' means the ability of the test to detect all the cases of Cystic Fibrosis among those tested. 'Specificity' means the ability to give a normal test result in all those who do not have Cystic Fibrosis.

The diagnosis will have been suggested by one or more of the symptoms already described, and the single most important diagnostic procedure is the Sweat Test. In this harmless and painless test, a small area of skin is stimulated to produce sweat which is collected on filter paper and the amount of salt (sodium and chloride) measured. Normal children have sweat concentrations for both chloride and sodium below 40 units (mmol/l): children with Cystic Fibrosis have values well over this—60–140 units; most cases 80–120. It is essential that the test should be carried out in a centre accustomed to regular sweat testing, with quality control monitoring, and a sound data bank of normal values. The sweat salt abnormality of Cystic Fibrosis is present at birth, affects almost 100 per cent of patients and persists throughout life.

One positive sweat test does not by itself establish the diagnosis and a repeat test is essential to confirm the diagnosis. There should also be some supporting factor, such as evidence of some degree of pancreatic deficiency, or chronic or recurrent bronchial or lung trouble, or a positive family history of Cystic Fibrosis. X-ray examination, various biochemical tests and sputum cultures may be required.

Prenatal Diagnosis

Parents of a Cystic Fibrosis child will have been told about the risks for further children, and the possibility of detecting during pregnancy whether the baby has Cystic Fibrosis. The research carried out at the University of Edinburgh by Professor Brook and his staff has made available a 95 per cent accurate diagnostic test for 'at risk' pregnancies. The test can be carried out at 17 to 18 weeks of gestation by taking a small sample of the amniotic fluid (which surrounds the baby in the womb) and measuring the level of certain enzymes.

Advances in genetic research now indicate the possibility of an accurate test by biopsy of the chorionic villus, which can be done at nine to 11 weeks. The family will decide whether to have the pregnancy terminated, which, by this test, can be done at three months.

Diagnosis at Birth: Screening

The practice of screening for important diseases (such as cervical cancer and high blood pressure) has developed in many countries in recent years. Newborn screening is widely performed in the United Kingdom for such conditions as thyroid deficiency and phenylketonuria, in which early diagnosis and treatment can have a markedly beneficial effect on the health and development of affected babies. In the case of Cystic Fibrosis there remain doubts and uncertainty regarding the value of newborn screening, and the results of controlled trials, such as that in progress in Wales and the West Midlands, are awaited with great interest. Newborn screening for Cystic Fibrosis is in fact carried out in a number of regions in the United Kingdom and EEC countries. The author was involved in the procedure over 25 years and recently reviewed the results in nearly four million screening tests. See the Table on p. 26.

'Screening' is carried out by means of a painless and harmless test which sorts out those babies who are probably Cystic Fibrosis from those who are probably not. Screening tests are not intended to be finally diagnostic, and positive tests must be confirmed and followed, with the least possible delay, by one or more specific diagnostic tests, together with full clinical evaluation. Of the many and various screening tests developed over the years, most have been found wanting and discarded; a few have been modified and are still used.

There is, however, general agreement that the best newborn screening test at present available is the Immunoreactive Trypsin test (IRT) which uses the dried blood spot collection from all newborns for the conditions previously mentioned. About 300 babies with Cystic Fibrosis are born each year in the United Kingdom. One of the arguments advanced in favour of newborn screening is based on the fact that in Cystic Fibrosis babies the lungs are virtually normal at birth, so that preventive treatment, including physiotherapy, can be started at once; this should prevent or mitigate the chronic broncho-pulmonary disease which is the major cause of disability and untimely death. The relatively better outlook for those Cystic Fibrosis babies born with meconium ileus also suggests a benefit from the earliest possible diagnosis and immediate medical and social care.

DIAGNOSIS OF CYSTIC FIBROSIS AT BIRTH: NEWBORN SCREENING

Tests on Newborn Bowel Motions—Meconium

TYPE OF TEST	NUMBER	CF FOUND	SENSITIVE	SPECIFIC
Traditional BM	1,738,794	601	79%	99.5%
Immunological	784,866	208	81%	99.0%
Electro-Immune	1,586,597	441	78%	99.5%
Total	4,110,257	1,250		

Newborn Blood Test (IRT)

ORIGIN OF TEST	NUMBER	CF FOUND	SENSITIVE	SPECIFIC
Europe	125,239	44	100%*	99.9%
USA/Canada	190,650	74	100%*	99.9%
United Kingdom	138,523	53	100%*	99.9%
Total	454,412	171	*1 false neg.	

Diagnostic Counselling

When the results of all the tests and investigations have been collected, a full diagnostic picture of the case can be assembled, and a meeting arranged with members of the medical team (doctor, nurse, physiotherapist, dietician) and both parents—it is important that at first, anyway, the father should be there. Parents may rightly expect the doctors to be competent and thorough—honest in answering questions, truthful, patient and understanding. Doctors and other members of the medical team will want the parents (and the patient) to co-operate as fully as possible: to learn about Cystic Fibrosis, ask questions, practise physiotherapy and become adept at their part in the management at home.

First, they must come to express their feelings on learning the diagnosis of Cystic Fibrosis; secondly, with help from the medical team, they must come to understand how they feel as they do; last, they will learn gradually how to cope with their feelings and the changed family situation, and to adapt and adjust to the overall plan of management.

Immediate shock, experienced by all parents on hearing the diagnosis, is quickly followed by a sort of 'mourning' reaction, with feelings of grief; also guilt and shame in many cases, when the hereditary nature of Cystic Fibrosis is first encountered. Other feelings commonly described are helplessness, futility and anxiety in varying degree of intensity. Doctors in particular must appreciate that while they can measure such things as pancreatic enzymes, blood oxygen levels, fat absorption, etc., in accurate scientific terms (milligrammes, millimols, pH, etc.), there are no equivalent measurements for the emotions, no pH for grief, no millimols for anxiety, depression or even hope. These emotional experiences can only be assayed subjectively, by the person experiencing them. Quite often, and nearly always with mothers, the anxiety experienced, accompanied by depression, makes it difficult to attend to the discussions about Cystic Fibrosis; it may impair their judgement and, for a time, limit their active participation in the treatment. Some may appear querulous, demanding and 'difficult', projecting blame on the husband or the doctor. Some may say, 'I must be stupid. I followed all you told me about Cystic Fibrosis, but I just can't seem to take it in.' All this, coming from an intelligent young woman who has just answered correctly all the factual questions put by the doctor, yet shows in her statements and behaviour that she seems not to believe her child has Cystic Fibrosis at all, can be puzzling and irritating to some people.

This in fact is characteristic of a well recognised mental process termed 'denial', a defence mechanism whereby the mother registers the doctor's facts in her mind but does not acknowledge their significance for the future. So denial is common and helpful: it will pass, especially as the family learns to cope and adjust, to take an active part in treatment, and the mother can feel that there is hope after all. What is needed from those around her is not confrontation —'face the facts'—but patient and understanding support.

Occasionally, on learning the diagnosis, a mother will express feelings of relief: 'I knew there was something seriously wrong with him all the time; I thought it might be cancer.' This is more common if the 'pre-diagnostic phase' has been characterised by considerable and continuous distress.

The Pre-Diagnostic Phase
This may be defined as the interval between the parents' first fears about the child's health and the day when the diagnosis of Cystic Fibrosis is disclosed to them. In one series studied in Europe, in 30 per cent of cases the diagnosis was made within three months of the first suspicion that 'something was wrong': in just over half of the cases this suspicion occurred during the first months of life. In a further 35 per cent the diagnosis was made before 12 months had elapsed after suspicion had first been aroused. The pre-diagnostic period can be very distressing: mothers blame themselves for some imagined shortcomings in child rearing. Neighbours and the extended family are not always helpful, indeed often critical, and maternal

depression is common. As one mother said, 'I could not enjoy my child for one minute.'

Accurate Diagnosis
Clearly, this is mandatory: if the requisites previously mentioned (two properly done sweat tests, evidence of pancreatic malfunction and intestinal malabsorption, some pointer to chest involvement, possibly family history) are followed, mistakes should not occur and in fact are very rarely reported today, compared with ten years ago. Missed cases (false negative diagnosis) lead to psychosocial stress like that experienced in a long pre-diagnostic phase, and when eventually corrected produce a severely traumatic situation for all concerned. Maternal resentment, anger, bitterness and depression are common. Sometimes, again, there is also a feeling of relief: 'I knew all along he had something.'

False positive diagnosis, when put right, leads to a different psychosocial situation: mixed with relief there is initial disbelief; often, surprisingly, depression and reluctance to give up the over-protective super-bonding relationship between mother and child which had become established. Family cohesion is disturbed. As one father put it, 'The footprints of Cystic Fibrosis are still around in this home.'

4 MANAGEMENT OF CYSTIC FIBROSIS

The strategic aim for Cystic Fibrosis patients is to help them reach adulthood with controlled physical disability and a psychosocial adaptation which allows them a nearly normal life-style, with minimal dependency. Ultimately, patients should be able to look after their own health, and to develop their potential assets towards an appropriate career, social life and marriage. This concept of self-advocacy must run throughout the whole course of management, from infancy through childhood and adolescence, resulting in a mature person who is a contributing member of the community. At the present time, with 'optimal care', some 70 to 80 per cent of Cystic Fibrosis patients may look forward to achieving these aims. Future prospects hold out the hope of even better results.

How are we to set about attaining these goals? It cannot be done by the doctors on their own; nor by the unaided devoted care of parents and family; nor by government services or charitable institutions by themselves—though each and all of these are required in the context of total care.

The essential requirement is a planned scheme of 'shared caring', tailored to individual cases and put into action as soon as the diagnosis of Cystic Fibrosis is made. The lynchpin of the scheme in the general management and specialised therapy is the establishment of close co-operation and understanding between the parents (and the patients as they grow and develop) and the medical team. The main components are:

1 Early, accurate diagnosis.
2 Initial hospitalisation for:
   a) Full evaluation ('diagnosis in depth').
   b) Intensive treatment of any existing lung disease.

c) Establishing the family/medical 'Action Group'—
by conveying information about Cystic Fibrosis in
general, and particularly with regard to the patient:
explaining what the medical team has to offer and
educating and training the family in shared home
care. The psychosocial effects of long term illness
such as Cystic Fibrosis form an important part of
this.

d) Preparing for discharge home, and the setting up of
techniques and equipment.

e) Home care, with regular out-patient and domicili-
ary follow-up.

3 Aspects requiring special detailed review:

a) The Respiratory System: including preventive measures, treatment of infections, physiotherapy, the
value of physical exercise.

b) Diet and Nutrition.

c) Schooling and further education and training.

d) Special problems of Adolescence.

e) Jobs and Careers.

Initial Treatment and Assessment

No apology is necessary for re-emphasising the prime
importance in Cystic Fibrosis of the health of the whole
respiratory tract, from nose and throat down the air tubes to
the lungs. It is this which exerts a 90 per cent influence on
the length and quality of your child's life.

The lungs, when examined at birth, seem virtually
normal, although minute microscopical examination
may show that the mucus-secreting glands in the walls
of the bronchial tubes appear enlarged. We know that the
bronchial secretions they produce are abnormally thick and
sticky, tending to block the tubes and impair the normal
clearing mechanisms of the lungs. Thus, infection easily
occurs, usually quite early in life. The bacteria found are not
the usual germs of adult pneumonia (pneumococcus): the
earliest invader is the staphylococcus, the common cause of
pustules, boils, carbuncles and other skin infections; a
bacterium belonging to the pseudomonas family has been

increasingly common over the past two decades, usually in older children, but in some cases also in infants.

When a child first comes into the Cystic Fibrosis unit for a full evaluation, the respiratory tract is examined clinically, by X-ray, and by some lung function tests appropriate for his age. Sputum cultures are very important, showing not only the presence of bacteria but also the type of organism, as well as sensitivity tests to indicate the best antibiotics to be used.

The first task, then, is the intensive treatment of any chest infection found. Increasingly powerful antibiotics are available, effective against the organisms mentioned, which can be given by intravenous infusion to even the smallest child. The bronchial obstructive element, due to the viscosity of the secretions, also requires treatment by frequent expert physiotherapy, with postural drainage. In some centres, aerosol inhalation treatment is added, using substances to make the mucus less sticky, or to open up the bronchial tubes; antibiotics may also be given by aerosol. The 'mist tents' which were widely used at one time have been shown to have defects and some hazards, and are no longer advocated. This use of intensive treatment, with appropriate intravenous antibiotics and intensive physio-therapy, has been shown in many cases to reverse the symptoms, also the signs in the chest and X-ray changes.

When the lung infection has been controlled and the child's general condition has improved, the parents (who have been studying and practising physiotherapy and other treatments) can be permitted to carry out the therapy on their own child, under direct supervision. When their instruction is complete and they are judged capable, and are confident about their ability to treat their child ad-equately, preparations for discharge and the home care programme can begin.

There are three common infections which affect the lungs, and would be very likely to aggravate the situation in a child with Cystic Fibrosis. They are Whooping Cough, Measles and Influenza. Immunisation against these is safe and effective, with the usual proper precautions, and should be carried out for Cystic Fibrosis children at the appropriate ages.

Next in importance, after the lungs, in the initial assessment of the patient, comes the evaluation of nutrition, digestion and absorption; also growth and development. With the onset of respiratory symptoms the traditional good appetite of the Cystic Fibrosis child begins to fade away, so insufficient intake of nourishment is added to the digestive problems. Also, nutrition and lung infections are linked, so that worsening of the one can affect the other; conversely, clearing up the chest improves nutrition; while better dietary manipulation plus modern pancreatic extract treatment will improve the child's ability to resist and combat the broncho-pulmonary infection.

In addition to the routine measurements of weight, height and head circumference, various blood and biochemical tests are made, and notes taken on bone development, pancreatic function and food absorption.

The Shared-Care Team

During the time of preparation for shared home care, small groups of parents of patients in the Cystic Fibrosis unit, after their session of practical work with nurses, physiotherapist and dietician, sit down with the medical people for a 'teach-in'. The knowledge of Cystic Fibrosis that has been attained is assessed, and parents are encouraged to ask questions and make comments.

On one occasion a father said, 'You have told us the great importance of preventing lung damage if possible, and how vaccination against Whooping Cough, Measles and Influenza can help in this direction. You have also told us, and it is in the reading notes you provided, that the lungs are virtually normal at birth in Cystic Fibrosis, and that infection occurs early in life. In addition, you have said that it is now possible to diagnose Cystic Fibrosis in newborn babies by a relatively simple and inexpensive blood-spot test. Why, then, don't you diagnose all Cystic Fibrosis babies at birth and give them appropriate antibiotic treatment to prevent lung damage?'

The answer to this question cannot be given shortly, for there are many factors involved. The health of the lungs is of prime importance for the future of the Cystic Fibrosis child, for it is the degree of chronic progressive bronchopulmonary infection and lung damage which determines how he will thrive. It is true also that at birth the lungs are virtually normal, but the as yet unknown basic defect of Cystic Fibrosis leads to the production of abnormally viscous bronchial mucus secretions which block the bronchial tubes, partially or completely, and impair the normal clearance mechanism of the lungs. We are always breathing into our lungs, not only air itself, but various microscopical particles, including dusts, smog, tobacco smoke and various bacteria. Normally these particles are subsequently swept along by ciliary action and air currents, including coughing, towards the throat, and are expelled. In Cystic Fibrosis this does not happen, so colonisation of the respiratory tract by bacteria occurs more easily. Colonisation precedes infection, and as the bacteria multiply, they invade and damage the tissues. This begins early in life, often in the first few months. Preventive measures are obviously highly desirable, if they can be shown to be both effective and without harmful side effects.

As I have said, it is possible to diagnose Cystic Fibrosis in newborn infants by the immunoreactive trypsin test (IRT), carried out in a regional laboratory using the blood spots taken at birth on all infants. The test is accurate, sensitive and specific and initial positive screening tests are confirmed by a repeat test two or three weeks later; the full diagnosis of Cystic Fibrosis is then completed by sweat testing, followed by the additional investigations previously described. So it should be possible eventually to detect annually in the United Kingdom some 300–400 Cystic Fibrosis babies shortly after birth. What then?

Deciding on a Treatment Programme

The First Option
Continuous preventive antibiotic treatment to all detected Cystic Fibrosis infants would be the obvious choice. In practice this would almost invariably mean anti-staphylococcal drugs, as this organism is nearly always the first invader. Parents should be acquainted with the names of antibiotics most commonly used in this situation, as the drugs would continue to be administered by them at home. Most Cystic Fibrosis centres using this antibiotic preventive therapy employ Flucloxacillin (sometimes combined with another antibiotic such as Amoxycillin or Erythromycin). Flucloxacillin is given by mouth (orally), usually as Floxapen Syrup, (one 5 ml teaspoon dose, when reconstituted with water, equals 125 mg) every six hours at least 30 minutes before any feed. This dose is prescribed for infants up to one year old: if the treatment is to be continued beyond this age the dose is doubled (250 mg).

Should infection occur, the choice of antibiotic depends, of course, upon the results of bacteriological tests on cough swabs, which would be taken at regular intervals.

There is at present no consensus of opinion regarding the advisability of long term preventive antibiotic treatment. Some authorities have been concerned that it could lead to other bacteria (pseudomonas, haemophilus, klebsiella) getting into the lungs, but there is no conclusive evidence for this. In any case, it is important to eradicate staphylococcus from the lungs and in Flucloxacillin-resistant cases, claims have been advanced for the efficacy of a combination treatment with Clindamycin and Fucidin.

The Second Option
Even without continuous antibiotic treatment, diagnosis very soon after birth confers other benefits. First, the parents are aware of their problem from the start and the problems of the pre-diagnostic phase do not bother them. Then again, bearing in mind the mutual relationship between lung infection and nutrition, early diagnosis allows

the nutritional state, feeding and dietary requirements to receive full attention so that the child can cope with respiratory bacteria. The state of the lungs is checked and closely monitored, including cough swab cultures at frequent intervals, with an intensive approach to the appearance of potential respiratory damaging bacteria.

Assuming that regular hospital and perhaps home follow-up visits and appropriate examinations are carried out, this option is favoured by many consultants, using intensive intravenous therapy when the situation demands. Antibiotics employed against the dangerous 'pseudomonas' group include Gentamycin, Azlocillin, Carbenicillin and Ceftazidime. Two-fold combinations of anti-pseudomonal drugs are usually employed (Ceftazidime with Gentamycin is a powerful treatment) by intravenous infusion over a period of two to three weeks, under close observation and guided by bacteriological and sensitivity tests.

This treatment necessitates admission to hospital, certainly at first. It is now possible for short courses of intravenous antibiotic treatment to be administered at home, using apparatus such as Port-a-Cath, or Venflon. Parents need to know the names and dosage of the drugs used; in suitable cases they will be taught the care and maintenance of the equipment, and those who successfully engage in home intravenous therapy gain increased self-esteem, while the patient gains in health and independence. The scheme has been used for children over six years of age. Co-operation with and monitoring by the hospital team are essential: a nurse pays home visits and takes serum samples on the third day of treatment, for the laboratory to check the blood concentration of the antibiotics.

Reports of the organisation and running of home intravenous antibiotic treatment from the United Kingdom, Europe and America are generally favourable. Older children appreciate the programme, which enables school work to be carried on, and they feel able to carry on their ordinary lives in most respects. Antibiotics have also been successfully administered by inhalation; good results are reported using a combination of Gentamycin and Carbenicillin, with a suitable machine.

Finally, an anti-pseudomonal antibiotic has recently been introduced which is effective when given by mouth. Ciprofloxacin, orally, has been shown to be a useful short term treatment for patients with Cystic Fibrosis who are infected with the aeruginosa strain of the pseudomonas germ.

Ciprofloxacin is a compound which was found in laboratory tests to be highly effective against pseudomonas, which is undoubtedly, the most troublesome infecting agent in the respiratory tract of Cystic Fibrosis patients, especially during later childhood and adolescence. The antibiotics described above are capable of controlling, though not completely eradicating, this organism from the lungs; they frequently require two to three weeks of intravenous therapy, repeated every three to four months. The introduction of home intravenous therapy certainly reduces the stress and strain of these otherwise essential hospitalisations, but home therapy is not widely applicable as yet. Ciprofloxacin, effective when given orally in a dosage averaging 500 mg, three times daily for six weeks, has reduced the necessity for frequent hospital admission and so far promises to be a valuable adjunct in treatment.

Ancillary Therapy
It is important to remember that in Cystic Fibrosis respiratory tract therapy, antibiotics alone are not enough. Best results are obtained when physiotherapy and breathing exercises, suited to the patient's age, are combined with antibiotic treatment, and when the optimum nutritional health is maintained by diet and pancreatic enzyme replacement medication.

To sum up, when considering how best to plan for the Cystic Fibrosis baby diagnosed soon after birth, there would appear at first sight to be two options:

1 Continuous preventive antibiotic treatment with Flucloxacillin or some other anti-staphylococcal antibiotic,

started at diagnosis and maintained permanently. Should infection by other bacteria (not sensitive to the continuous antibiotic) occur, intermittent treatment by additional appropriate antibiotics is given as required.

2 No continuous antibiotic treatment, but intermittent intensive treatment with appropriate antibiotics for any lung infections as they occur.

Informed opinion is at present equally divided regarding the respective merits of these treatments:

In favour of continuous therapy
The lungs are structurally normal at birth but especially liable to early infection with staphylococcus; there are some reported studies indicating that this can be controlled by the treatment.

Against continuous therapy
Prolonged continuous treatment can lead either to the appearance of resistant strains of staphylococcus or to infection by other, possibly more sinister bacteria which are not sensitive to the continuous antibiotic. There have been several reports of case studies supporting this objection, with particular reference to the pseudomonas group of organisms.

What is required to resolve this dilemma is a controlled trial on a fairly large scale, carried out by several centres in Europe and America. There would be two groups of Cystic Fibrosis babies diagnosed at birth. Management would be exactly the same for each group, apart from the giving or not giving of the continuous anti-staphylococcal antibiotic. One such trial is already underway between two centres in the United Kingdom and the results are eagerly awaited.

In the meantime, there is a practical compromise, based upon the stage of development of the lungs in the years from birth to five years. During this period the lungs are growing not only in volume but in complexity, with the development of new bronchial branches and the small lobes of the lungs to be served by these airways. These small, infantile airways are so easily blocked by the viscous Cystic Fibrosis mucus that the valuable, and indeed essential, physiotherapeutic techniques which are generally employed, are necessarily of limited application in this age group.

Compromise Treatment in Infancy

The treatment I would recommend, and which is practised in a number of Cystic Fibrosis clinics in the United Kingdom, is as follows:

1 Check that the chest is clear, and X-ray. Check that cough swabs grow no disease-causing bacteria (pathogens). If infection is found, give intensive treatment.

2 If the chest is found to be clear, begin preventive (prophylactic) medication with an anti-staphylococcal antibiotic such as Flucloxacillin; the dose and preparation will be written down for parents. The medicine is to be given on an empty stomach, say 30 minutes before meals. Some children find Flucloxacillin medicine bitter to the taste—one chocolate drop will not spoil their appetite!

3 Use physiotherapy, appropriate for age and development.

4 Regularly monitor the child's respiratory tract and general health, with visits to the local or central Cystic Fibrosis clinic, and home visits by nurses. These will include examinations, X-rays if necessary, and regular cough swabs for culture.

5 *Parent Watch.* We are familiar nowadays with the admirable Neighbourhood Watch and Child Watch schemes. In the Cystic Fibrosis context, doctors have found that parents (and older sisters or brothers) can play an equally active and useful part. The family is taught how to look out for symptoms which can indicate early lung infection: a change in the nature of the patient's cough, which may become more paroxysmal, loose or 'fruity', or lead to vomiting of thick mucus; unusual lethargy,

fretfulness, or loss of appetite; a rise in temperature, for while fever is not necessarily an early symptom—usually it comes later—any such indication would be very important; loss of weight.

One of the features of the shared care treatment must be the availability of the medical staff. Parents noting any of the symptoms just reviewed must have the right to contact a doctor without delay, so that further investigation and treatment can be arranged immediately. The importance of this, and the cough symptom in particular, cannot be over-rated.

PHYSIOTHERAPY

This is an essential part of the management of the respiratory tract in Cystic Fibrosis, being both preventive and curative. Physiotherapy aims at keeping the bronchial tubes as clear as possible, in order to facilitate the clearance of secretions out of the lungs and the entry of air into all the pulmonary segments. Efficient coughing is an important part of the techniques. Methods used include 'postural drainage', percussion (measured tapping) of the chest wall, manual vibration and shaking, followed by directed coughing and expectoration.

Postural drainage is based on the anatomy of the bronchial 'tree'. The patient is placed in each of five postures, so that gravity will assist drainage from each lung segment; the segment under attention is then treated by percussion (striking with the hands cupped) for about three minutes in each position, with vibrations and compression as necessary. Breathing exercises also form part of the sessions, which are done three to four times daily in hospital and twice daily, as a rule, at home. Proper diaphragmatic breathing (often neglected by people in general), is also taught and improves overall lung function. A recent and highly effective physiotherapy manoeuvre is the 'Forced Expiration Technique' which can be taught to children from about three years old. It is especially useful for adolescents and adults, enhancing not only their lung function but also their self-esteem and independence.

As mentioned previously, an important part of the educational programme for parents during the patient's initial hospitalisation is training in physiotherapy. Both parents should take part in this course of instruction, which will obviously include practice as well as theory. When they are felt to be competent, they may carry out the techniques appropriate for the patient's age under supervision in the hospital, and then continue at home. At a subsequent follow-up visit to the Cystic Fibrosis unit, they can demonstrate to the physiotherapist the techniques they use at home, as a check on their performance. In some centres, it is possible for home visits to be made by one of the physiotherapists, to help parents with any problems they may have with the treatment—such as timing the physiotherapy sessions to fit in with home routines, school, play and social life generally, and combining physiotherapy with nebulisation therapy, which has taken the place of the 'mist tents'.

Nebulisers
These are machines which convert a solution of a drug into an 'aerosol' mist by passing a fine high pressure air jet through the liquid. The mist may be inhaled via a face mask or a mouthpiece, breathing in slowly and deeply (expiration should be quicker as the aerosol is released continuously). The aim is to get as much of the drug as possible down into the smallest air passages, although some aerosol is inevitably deposited in the mouth and throat. Deep penetration of the aerosol depends upon using the correct breathing technique, the type of nebuliser and, most importantly, the size of the mist particles. There is a wide range of different-sized minute droplets in the mist, and tests using a radio-isotope technique show that particles of 1/5000 inch diameter or less are required to get right down to the lungs. With the best nebulisers, a high proportion of the drug reaches the lungs, rather than the nose, mouth and throat. The medical staff at the Cystic Fibrosis unit will

teach the correct use of the nebuliser and advise on care and maintenance of the equipment. The cost of the apparatus varies considerably, and again the doctors and technician will advise parents. It is sometimes possible to obtain a nebuliser on loan for an indefinite period under the National Health Service, if the consultant makes a recommendation. Inhalation treatment by nebuliser is used in several ways:

1 To loosen the phlegm—the medical term is 'mucolytic'. Drugs such as Airbron and Alevaire are sometimes prescribed to facilitate expectoration by reducing sputum viscosity. For children, 0.9 per cent saline solution acts as a moisturiser and helps to liquefy the clinging mucus, without the side effects that drugs may produce. Inhalation of 3 ml saline, given *before* postural drainage, is advised.

2 To relax spasm of the bronchial tubes (bronchodilators). Some Cystic Fibrosis babies and young children with chest infection may have wheezing and shortness of breath resembling Asthma: true Asthma may co-exist with Cystic Fibrosis, and similar symptoms occur when an unusual fungus (aspergillus) gains entry to the respiratory tract. Bronchospasm in those children liable to wheezing can sometimes occur during some of the physiotherapy manoeuvres involving forced breathing out, and during physical exercise, and the inhalation of an aerosol bronchodilator for ten minutes beforehand is advised. Either Salbutamol (Ventolin) or Terbutaline (Bricanyl), with saline, is suitable, to be given *before* physiotherapy.

3 Antibiotic nebulisation inhalation treatment has recently become more popular, as it has been proved not only to reduce symptoms generally, but to attain adequate levels in the blood, depending on the dose; also, the inhaled antibiotic can reach all parts of the lungs, even those not ventilated, via the blood, while inhalation into the ventilated parts exerts a noticeably beneficial local effect on the organisms producing infection. The treat-

ment, given at home after instruction, may also reduce the frequency of hospital admissions, providing the usual follow-up examinations and cough cultures are made.

The antibiotics used are:

Gentamycin (80 mg)
with
Carbenicillin (1 g)   } suspended in 2-4 ml saline

or

by nebulised inhalation twice daily

Tobramycin (80 mg)
with
Ticarcillin (1 g)   } suspended in 2-4 ml saline

These antibiotics are especially valuable in treating infection with pseudomonas.

Antibiotic inhalation treatment is given *after* physiotherapy has cleared the bronchial tubes.

Side Effects of Antibiotics
These are not very common and very seldom serious, but are unpleasant for patients already ill, and worrying for parents. It is important therefore to know the main reactions to different antibiotics so that parents may be able to detect the first symptoms and report to the medical team.

Penicillins (Pencillin G, Penicillin V, Cloxacillin, Flucloxacillin, Ampicillin, Azlocillin, Carbenicillin)
When given orally the penicillins may cause nausea, vomiting, and diarrhoea; sometimes, with diarrhoea, there is a painful irritating rash around the back passage after a few days. Oral antibiotics should be given on an empty stomach, say half an hour before meals. Important side effects are what is known as 'hypersensitivity reactions', resembling allergic conditions. These comprise rashes which can be very irritating, some of the 'nettlerash' type (urticaria), some resembling and easily mistaken for

measles. Occasionally the child has a sore mouth and the rash may be seen inside the cheeks. Other symptoms in this group are raised temperature, pain in various joints and puffiness of the face, especially around the eyes. It is very important for parents to report any reactions to penicillin which the child may have shown during previous treatment, since, although the first hypersensitivity reaction may not be severe, if penicillin is given subsequently the effects could be serious; if they are forewarned, the doctors can take appropriate steps.

Antibiotics Against Pseudomonas

Penicillins are best known for their use in the treatment of staphylococcal infection, but some later developed penicillins, such as Azlocillin and Carbenicillin, are used in conjunction with antibiotics of the Gentamycin group for the treatment of the very important pseudomonas lung infections. Azlocillin and Carbenicillin can give hypersensitivity reactions similar to Penicillin G.

The Gentamycin group (aminoglycosides) includes Gentamycin, Tobramycin, Netilmycin. They are useful and important drugs. Side effects are damage to the inner ear, which could lead to deafness, and to a lesser degree kidney damage. These side effects are most common in elderly patients but may also occur in children; they are dose-related, and if intravenous treatment with these antibiotics is organised at home, it is important for blood samples to be taken one hour after injection and also just before the next dose. The doses can then be regulated to keep the level of antibiotic in the blood within safe limits. (Neomycin by aerosol can cause deafness and this should not be used.)

Tetracyclines (e.g. Acromycin)

Acromycin, Aureomycin, Terramycin are broad-spectrum antibiotics useful in some cases of bronchial infection due to Haemophilus Influenzae. They can cause staining of developing teeth—at first a bright yellow colour which later darkens to brown. The psychosocial effects, especially in adolescence, can be severe, even though 'capping' and bleaching are sometimes tried. If possible, Tetracyclines should be avoided in children under the age of 12.

NUTRITIONAL MANAGEMENT
As regards nutrition generally in childhood, overall calorie supply is more important for a child's health than for an adult's. Children have relatively increased calorie needs (energy) compared with adults—for their basal metabolism, for activity, and above all for growth. In healthy children the appetite closely parallels the growth needs, so that young infants in their rapid growth period, and adolescents in their early teenage growth spurt, eat relatively more than they will a few years later, when growth rate has slowed down. Thus, the seven pound, full term baby needs 360 calories a day; at one year 1,000 calories, and the rapidly growing and developing 15-year-old needs about 3,000. Soldiers on active service, lumberjacks and other heavy workers need little more to maintain health and vigour.

These figures apply to healthy children, who digest and absorb their dietary nutriments. What, then, for the Cystic Fibrosis child, whose pancreas provides less than normal amounts of digestive enzymes, or none at all, with extra trouble in the intestine from mucus and depleted bile salts?

The traditional picture of the Cystic Fibrosis child is of one who fails to thrive—in spite of a large appetite and a good diet. With the onset of chest infections, early in life in most cases, the voracious appetite fails and malnutrition takes over. Slowing of weight gain shows first, then actual loss of weight, sometimes with added symptoms of deficiencies of vitamins, minerals and certain essential fatty acids. Lung infection both aggravates the nutritional problem and is itself aggravated by malnutrition. Slowing of growth in height shows later.

For many years the management of nutrition in Cystic Fibrosis comprised a low fat, high protein diet, combined with pancreatic enzyme preparations in powder, tablet or capsule form. Gastric acid can inactivate pancreatic enzymes, so a drug such as Cimetidine was given 45 minutes before the pancreatin (enzyme preparation) to inhibit temporarily the acid secretion, and so boost the action of the enzyme. This form of treatment was shown to increase the percentage absorption of ingested fat, to reduce the frequency of bowel movements and to improve their character. While there was some improvement in weight gain and growth, there was much variability in patients' response to the treatment, and it was rarely completely successful.

Recently there has been radical rethinking about nutrition in Cystic Fibrosis and its management by diet and enzyme replacement. This change of opinion has come about for two main reasons. First, the results of a number of studies and research programmes show that Cystic Fibrosis patients need a *much greater* nutritional intake (measured as calories) than normal children and adults—from one-and-a-quarter to one-and-a-half times the normal daily food allowance for health (the official term is 'Recommended Daily Allowances'—RDA—used by the DoH in the United Kingdom and the NRC in the United States). This extra requirement is needed because, due to pancreatic enzyme deficiency and intestinal malabsorption, the Cystic Fibrosis patient loses a significant amount of food intake in the frequent bulky, greasy stools. Extra energy from food is also needed to combat lung infection. In addition, the 'Resting Energy Requirement' has been found by research workers to be higher than normal in Cystic Fibrosis. Dietary fat provides twice as many calories, weight for weight, as protein or carbohydrate, essential as these nutrients are.

The second reason for the new thinking is the introduction of more effective pancreatic enzyme preparations. The older powders and tablets raised the fat absorption to a certain extent, but 80–90 per cent fat absorption can now be effected by giving the newer enteric coated microspheres —for example, Creon or Pancrease. These microspheres contain protease, amylase and lipase, for the digestion of protein, carbohydrate and fat respectively. They are enclosed in a gelatin capsule which dissolves in the stomach, releasing the microspheres which are protected from the acid peptic gastric juice by a special coating. This dissolves only in the small intestine, thus releasing the enzymes intact where they are needed. So fat as a major source of energy is now possible in the Cystic Fibrosis diet, without unpleasant abdominal symptoms, but with good nutritional effect. Some patients have some residual pancreatic function, during early childhood anyway, and have had good nutritional results with some of the older enzyme preparations such as Pancrex, Nutrizym and Cotazym; they may continue with these unless pancreatic function deteriorates further with the passage of time.

The capsules containing the new microspheres may be swallowed whole during each meal, or may be opened and the microspheres taken with a little liquid. They should never be added to food being prepared for cooking, or to hot meals. The actual dose to be used will vary for each individual patient, depending on the bowel motions and weight gain.

*   *   *

So far this section has dealt with the main outlines of nutritional strategy for Cystic Fibrosis. Parents will want to know what foods suitable for children contain adequate amounts of protein, or fat, or carbohydrates and vitamins. A general answer can be given here, but I must emphasise the prime importance, in this context, of close family liaison with a qualified dietician who will give detailed information on food values, selection and preparation of main meals and the essential snacks which children love and which can be made a valuable nutritional supplement. She will also help in regular dietary monitoring.

The principal protein-providing foods are meat, fish and poultry; vegetables, cereals and nuts also provide useful protein. Dairy foods such as milk, cheese, yoghurt and eggs are convenient sources of first class protein which can be prepared and presented in a variety of appetising dishes.

Carbohydrates include the starchy foods such as bread, biscuits, cereals, rice, potatoes, pasta, flour, and noodles; sugars include white and brown cane sugar, syrup, treacle, sweets, sweet biscuits and cakes, squashes, fruit and most fizzy drinks. Cows' milk contains four per cent milk sugar (lactose). Fats are provided by butter, margarine, cream, ice-cream, chocolate, pastry, fried food and potato crisps. In some cases a special, easily absorbed fat known as MCT (medium-chain triglyceride) is advised. It is usually used as an oil in cooking.

In addition to three meals daily, there is a case for supplementary feeding to bring the total daily energy supply up to the desired level. Supplements are most conveniently given as snacks between meals, in the form of high protein, high energy drinks. Strawberry Milk Shake, Build-up Milk Shake and Chocolate Cooler, for example, provide 200–400 calories a time. Recipes for these and other mouth-watering energising preparations will be given by the dietician; they are also provided, together with a great deal of practical nutritional information and advice, in the excellent booklet *Nutritional Management of Cystic Fibrosis*, obtainable from the Cystic Fibrosis Research Trust. Full details of this admirable institution are given in Chapter Twelve.

Vitamin Supplements
Vitamins A, D, E and K are the fat-soluble micronutrients and therefore liable to be involved in the fat malabsorption and loss of fat in the bowel motions which characterise Cystic Fibrosis. Natural sources of vitamins in the diet are therefore doubtfully reliable and vitamin supplements are considered advisable.

Vitamin A is found in liver, milk and dairy produce, egg yolk and carrots. Deficiency in this vitamin affects growth, may cause eye disease (night blindness is a symptom), and dry scaly changes in the skin and cell lining of the bronchial tubes; rarely, it may lead to raised pressure within the skull of the newborn baby.

Vitamin D is essential for the proper calcification of bone, and deficiency results in rickets in children and osteoporosis in adults. In health, the vitamin is ingested in fish oil, also produced in the skin by the action of sunlight.

Vitamin E is present in vegetables and seed oils. Deficiency symptoms are not common in Cystic Fibrosis, even though blood levels are often found to be low; some reports indicate cases of an unusual type of anaemia; neuromuscular disorders have also been implicated.

Vitamin K (dietary sources include green leafy vegetables, butter and liver) is necessary for the production of blood clotting factors, also certain proteins for normal bone development. Cystic Fibrosis babies are prone to Vitamin K deficiency, leading to haemorrhagic symptoms ranging from easy bruising to frank bleeding, necessitating hospital treatment.

Regular daily supplements of the fat soluble vitamins are therefore advised for all Cystic Fibrosis patients. The doctor will advise and prescribe suitable preparations for all ages. Deficiencies of water soluble vitamins, the C and B groups, are not known to occur in Cystic Fibrosis.

Minerals

There is as yet no general consensus of opinion regarding the need for dietary supplementation of minerals such as iron, copper, zinc, and selenium. A recent report indicated low blood iron, copper, zinc, and selenium. A recent report indicated low blood iron levels in one third of Cystic Fibrosis patients studied, but no gross anaemia. It would probably be wise periodically to check the blood count and iron, but regular daily doses are not advised. Copper, zinc and selenium function as the activating force in various enzymes and some reports indicate low blood levels in cases of Cystic Fibrosis. There is no hard evidence on this, and further investigations are in progress. Certainly, no dietary supplementation is recommended at present.

With regard to salt, which is present in excessive amounts in the sweat, the consequences of sodium or salt depletion in Cystic Fibrosis patients can be catastrophic in hot climates or during heat waves, when exposure and/or physical exertion causes increased sweating, with dehydration, salt depletion and shock. If Cystic Fibrosis patients have to be in hot environments and exposed to the sun, with physical activity, and therefore increased sweating, then salt tablets are required. The dose and its frequency will be determined by the doctors at the time and place.

Infant Feeding for Cystic Fibrosis
As stated at the beginning of this section, small infants need a relatively large amount of food, of high energy content and containing adequate amounts of first class protein. The basis of infant feeding is milk. This may be breast milk, cows' milk (or both), some form of modified or fortified cows' milk, or Pregestimil, a synthetic milk composed of glucose, predigested milk protein, corn oil, apricot starch, MCT (medium-chain triglyceride) and minerals.

Breast milk has certain advantages over cows' milk: both provide 20 calories per ounce, but in breast milk the proteins are more easily digested, the fat more finely emulsified and therefore more easily absorbed, and the milk sugar (lactose) content is much higher. The mother's milk also contains Vitamins A, B, C and D, together with minerals appropriate for a small baby's needs; finally, there are some antibacterial and antiviral compounds.

Artificial feeding by bottle may have to be done, using a modified cows' milk such as SMA Gold Cap or Cow & Gate Premium. Both these excellent products may be fortified if necessary by skimmed milk powder, and glucose powders such as Polycal, Caloreen or Maxijul. Pancreatin has to be given before bottle or breast feeds—for example, the contents of one capsule of Cotazym with a little milk from spoon or syringe; never put it into the bottle.

Pregestimil has been shown to promote growth and weight gain in small Cystic Fibrosis babies who were weak and ill, some having had surgical operations in the newborn period. One group in the United States, followed for 12 months, achieved normal figures for weight and length.

For the 'well' Cystic Fibrosis infant, who takes the breast

or bottle easily and can ingest the increased food requirements that the disease enforces, such special feeds are
unnecessary. The average British newborn infant of seven-
and-a-half pounds weight requires 360 calories per day;
that means seven milk feeds averaging two-and-a-half
ounces each. The Cystic Fibrosis infant of the same weight
needs at least 440 calories daily, or seven feeds, each over
three ounces. The Cystic Fibrosis milk formula described in
the Cystic Fibrosis Research Trust booklet supplies the high
energy, high protein milk feed needed by many babies.

I have no doubt that successful breast feeding has even
greater advantages than the biochemical superiority of the
milk. Its temperature, sterility and automatic feed adjustment are perfect, providing the baby is not too ill, weak or
premature to feed. The psychological uplift given by the
mother knowing and feeling that she is doing something
very positively beneficial for this Cystic Fibrosis baby she
has borne and delivered, goes a long way to assuage the
feelings of worry, depression and self-doubt which came
with the confrontation of the diagnosis. The unique physical contacts of breast feeding serve to reinforce the close
bonding with her baby that they both need, and so family
cohesion is promoted.

5 GENETICS AND THE CYSTIC FIBROSIS GENE

Human Genetics is that branch of medical science which deals with our heredity, the way in which we acquire some parts of our parents' attributes. These we do not inherit directly, but through a system of coded instructions stored in the nucleus of each of the myriad cells of the body. These coded messages are transmitted by the genes. Our genetic inheritance is all present in that particular egg cell in our mother after it is fertilised by our father's spermatozoon, at the moment of conception. The fertilised egg contains complete 'recipes' for growth and development of the foetus, infant and child, through adolescence to maturity.

Genes are therefore the basic units of inheritance. They are composed of a complex organic molecule usually referred to as DNA (Deoxyribonucleic acid); a gene is a code-bearing section of an awesomely long spiral thread of DNA carried in structures named chromosomes (see Figure 1, p. 12) which are present only in the nucleus of a cell. Genes are arranged in linear fashion on the chromosomes and occupy definite positions (loci). Each cell in our bodies (except the sex cells—eggs and sperms) carries 46 chromosomes arranged in 23 pairs, one of the pair from the mother, the other from the father. In 22 pairs the chromosomes are the same kind (called autosomes): the 23rd pair are the sex-determining chromosomes, females having two large X chromosomes and males one large X and a small Y chromosome.

During the formation of the reproductive cells the number of chromosomes in each cell becomes halved (23): the mother's eggs all carry an X, the father's sperms are half X carriers and half Y carriers. The fertilised egg contains all the sperm's genetic information as well, so has 46 chromosomes; therefore so have the cells of the developing embryo.

Geneticists estimate that between two and two-and-a-half million men and women in Britain carry the defective gene which causes Cystic Fibrosis. Progress in this area of genetics has been made by co-operative studies in several countries, including Professor Williamson's group at St Mary's Hospital Medical School, and other centres in Britain. The Cystic Fibrosis gene has been located at a site on the long arm of Chromosome 7; work continues towards isolation of the gene and discovery of the gene product.

We can now follow the genetic sequence leading to a Cystic Fibrosis baby (see Figure 1). Each parent is a heterozygote carrier of the abnormal Cystic Fibrosis gene at the specific locus on the long arm of one of their pair of Chromosomes No. 7. At the same locus on the other chromosome of their pair there is a normal gene, which is dominant, so that it gets the job done; the single Cystic Fibrosis gene, being recessive, is not expressed. Each parent is therefore quite healthy (in fact they could just possibly possess some as yet undiscovered biological advantage).

The genes on the chromosomes in the nucleus of the cell dominate cell life and metabolic activity by controlling the production of numerous building-block type proteins, and also enzymes which regulate the numerous activities of our bodies.

We do not yet know what particular building protein or enzyme the gene at the Cystic Fibrosis locus on Chromosome No. 7 is responsible for programming. The basic defect in Cystic Fibrosis could be due either to the effects of deficiency of that protein or to the abnormal production of some variant which adversely affects various secretions: possibly a combination of both. With the heterozygotes (the parents), however, the dominant gene at the locus codes and programmes for the essential end product.

The father of one of my patients asked a very pertinent question about the genetics of Cystic Fibrosis.

'You have told us,' he said, 'that about 300 infants are

born with Cystic Fibrosis each year in the United Kingdom, and that some two-and-a-half million men and women in this country are carriers of the Cystic Fibrosis gene— apparently normal, healthy people. You have stated also that, until recently, comparatively few Cystic Fibrosis children survived to reproductive age, and in any case 98 per cent of Cystic Fibrosis males are infertile, and that successful pregnancy and delivery of a live child by a Cystic Fibrosis woman is comparatively uncommon. How, then, do you account for the persistence of this abnormal gene in people of the western world?'

He had evidently read up the subject of possible 'heterozygote advantage', and I was unable to supply a satisfactory answer, merely mentioning the possibilities of reproductive compensation, superior resistance to infections and cardiovascular disease, and gene mutation. None of these seems to experts a sufficient explanation.

He had a further question. 'How does your account of genetics explain the great natural variation in presentation and severity of this disease? You have related case histories showing that most patients are usually diagnosed early in life because of severe symptoms, but there are others who show a marked delay in the development of symptoms and escape detection until adolescence or even adult life.'

Again I could give no satisfactory explanation for the undoubted variation in severity and progression of Cystic Fibrosis, which has intrigued research workers on both sides of the Atlantic. One possibility is what is called 'genetic heterogeneity'. This means that there may be more than a single gene variant at the locus, or perhaps there are 'regulator' or modifying genes that alter the expression of the disease. Another explanation, put forward by American authorities, is that mutant genes at two separate sites (loci) are involved. Recent research suggests that the influence of regulator genes may be responsible for the variations (types) of Cystic Fibrosis, which clinical observers have found over a period of years.

The human body is made up of many millions of cells with varied shapes, sizes and functions but all having a similar basal structure. Cells are surrounded by a semi-permeable membrane which controls the entry and exit of many substances. Inside is a semi-fluid substance called 'cytoplasm', which serves as factory and store-house, and the vitally important nucleus which is what concerns us now. The nucleus is the control centre of the cell and contains the molecule we are most concerned with. This is the DNA (Deoxyribonucleic acid) which, in shape and form, looks like two intertwined spiral stairs. Each 'stair' is made up of a string of four basic molecules (you may think of them as a string of coloured beads: red, blue, green and yellow). These beads act as a sort of 'alphabet', and just like an ordinary alphabet, it is the order of the beads which conveys a message to the readers. In the cell the messages from the DNA are passed to units in the cytoplasm and transcribed into a sort of 'recipe' for the manufacture of numerous proteins and enzymes. 'Genes' are just the name given to particular lengths of bead sections of the DNA, and the message is read by the cell according to the order in which the beads are placed. Just as a misspelt word can make nansonse of what I am saying, so in the cell message a red bead where a blue ought to be, or a yellow left out altogether and two greens put in, can make nonsense of the genetic message to the cells.

In Cystic Fibrosis, a certain section of the string of beads which sends a message to the chemical factory in the cytoplasm has somehow got mixed up, so the lungs, the digestive organs and the sweat glands do not make one of the proper proteins which they require in order to function in a healthy manner.

The faulty arrangement of the beads in the Cystic Fibrosis gene could take the form of, 1) deletion of one or more of the component beads; 2) wrong order of beads; 3) insertion of an unwanted bead; 4) the beads the wrong way round; or there could be faulty 'copying' (transcribing) of the message. You can see how, in the heterozygote (carrier), the nonsense message is overruled by that coming from the dominant normal gene.

An everyday analogy would be in sending a recipe for

making a cake to a friend, via one or more messengers, who would copy it down (or remember it) incorrectly. The normal recipe would be:

Place in the mixer 8 oz self-raising flour, 3 eggs and 1 gill of milk.

I could get it wrong in several ways:

Place 8 oz flour and 3 eggs in 1 gill of milk.
Place 8 gills of milk and 3 oz flour in 1 egg.
Place 8 oz SR flour, 3 eggs and ½ cucumber in 1 gill milk.

You might get a cake of some kind out of one of these, but it certainly would not be the right one.

There are several other ways in which the gene message can become scrambled, which need not concern us here. My main point now is that we do not know which of these mix-ups results in the Cystic Fibrosis symptoms, nor do we yet know which function of the cell is disrupted by the abnormal gene action. Current molecular genetic research is well on the way to finding the answer.

In the following paragraphs I shall look at a number of situations and the questions arising from them, which I have encountered in my own clinical experience. As I have mentioned previously, the 'chances' that I give are statistically possible odds, which for the moment is the best we can do, apart from those 'informative' families known to the geneticists. The availability for an accurate diagnostic test to detect heterozygote Cystic Fibrosis carriers will greatly clarify the situation.

I advise parents, patients and families to keep in touch with their genetic counsellors, and not hesitate to ask repeatedly for the situation to be explained until they are quite clear in their minds.

Question
My brother has Cystic Fibrosis. I am quite well and healthy; I had a sweat test when my brother was diagnosed and it

was normal. I'm engaged to be married and I've told my girl about the Cystic Fibrosis; there's none in her family, she said. What chance is there that we could have a Cystic Fibrosis baby?

Answer
Both your parents must be carriers, so there is a ⅔ chance that you could be a carrier. Your wife will have the usual estimated carrier chance of 1/25, so the theoretical statistical chance that you are both carriers is 2/3 × 1/25 = 2/75, and the chance that your baby would be Cystic Fibrosis is 2/3 × 2/25 × 1/4 = 1/150; 1 in 150 is not highly probable—the odds are 149 to one against. Of course, if your wife is not a carrier, even if you are, then there would be no chance of having a Cystic Fibrosis baby.

Question
I've been married for just over a year now. We are thinking about starting a family and would like to have your advice. You see, my brother's wife has just had her first baby and he had to have an operation soon after he was born, because of some obstruction of the bowels. They did some tests on him and the specialist told my sister-in-law the baby had Cystic Fibrosis. She read in a book that this was hereditary and can run in the family. What are the chances I might have a baby with Cystic Fibrosis? Is there any way of finding out? There's nothing like it in my husband's family.

Answer
Your brother must be a carrier, and one at least of your parents. It is theoretically possible that your other parent is a carrier too, in which case you would have a one in two chance of being a carrier also. Your husband has a one in 25 chance, so the possibility that you are both carriers is 1/2 × 1/25 = 1/50; and the risk of having a Cystic Fibrosis baby is therefore 1/4 × 1/50 = 1/200, the odds being 199 to one against. If your husband is not a carrier, even if you are, then there is no risk.

Question
I should be grateful for advice regarding a possible pregnancy. This is my second marriage. My first husband was killed in a road accident, leaving me with a year-old baby boy. The child was delicate, with a chronic cough and several attacks of pneumonia. He was diagnosed as CF at the age of two-and-a-half, when he was in hospital with one of these chest infections, and he died just after his third birthday. I am now 31 and both my second husband and myself would like to have a child, but I am rather afraid it could turn out to be CF again. Is this possible, or am I worrying unnecessarily? My husband is healthy and there is no history of Cystic Fibrosis in his family.

Answer
It depends whether your husband carries the Cystic Fibrosis gene or not. The chance of this is 1 in 25. If he is not a carrier (you should realise that you must be one) then there is no chance of you having a Cystic Fibrosis child, although half your offspring would be carriers. If your husband is a carrier, the risk of you having a Cystic Fibrosis child would be $1/25 \times 1/4 = 1/100$, that is 99 to one against.

6   THE IMPACT OF CYSTIC FIBROSIS ON THE FAMILY

Since the recognition of Cystic Fibrosis half a century ago, knowledge and management has progressed so that the outlook for early diagnosed patients is now greatly improved. The parents have come to know about the inheritance of the disease, what goes wrong in various parts of the patient's body, what symptoms are shown, and how the diagnosis is made. Then they have come to learn about the management and medical treatment, in which they will play an important part at home with the patient. This will involve twice daily physiotherapy and breathing exercises, administration of antibiotics and other medicines, organising and checking food intake and supplements, as well as the usual routines of caring for a young child and promoting his overall well-being and happiness. 'Some task!' you may well say.

We now have to recognise that in Cystic Fibrosis, as in other long-term handicapping disorders, the impact of the diagnosis upon the family, followed by the necessary adjustments in family life and adaptation to the changed situation, can induce stress which may lead to problems of an emotional and psychological nature. These are just as important as the physical symptoms and need just as careful handling. In the same way that we set out to prevent, if possible, and certainly to lessen, the severity of lung infections, so we have to try to prevent and minimise family stress reactions which could impair the comprehensive care programme of the 'whole child'. Again, just as the physical symptoms of Cystic Fibrosis vary from case to case in variety and severity, so do the emotional and psychological problems. *Long term care of the Cystic Fibrosis child by no means invariably leads to severe disturbance in the life of that family.*

In this chapter we shall look at the various psychosocial problems which may occur in families, beginning with those affecting the mother, father and Cystic Fibrosis child, and going on to discuss the effects on brothers and sisters, grandparents and other relatives. Lastly, we shall consider the interreactions with the caring people who will be in regular contact: the doctors, health workers, social services personnel, as well as friends and neighbours and the local community. Suggested methods for minimising the problems are described.

The Effect on the Family

The Mother's 'Denial' and the Doctor's Truth

Learning that her child has an incurable inherited disease confronts his mother immediately with shock and stress, grief, anxiety and worry. Then she learns what Cystic Fibrosis means to the patient, with the promise that her child will reach adulthood but with varying degrees of disability and the likelihood of recurring complications. She learns gradually what is expected of her in the care of her child, and of the alterations required in her life and that of her husband. This is where the psychic defence mechanism termed 'denial' comes in. It enables her to register the medical facts of the case as explained by the medical team, and to answer the doctor's questions better than anyone else in the family group, so that they say, 'she knows it all'; but her 'denial' means that she only absorbs selective information: the implications of what she has heard and their ultimate meaning for the conduct of her child's life are not registered in her mind.

This is quite different from saying, 'I do not believe he has that dreadful disease. I want more tests done. I want another opinion.' The 'psychic denial' serves to preserve belief and hope, and in many cases it is necessary to enable the mother to continue mothering, nursing and bonding, and carrying on the various treatment schedules at home, with regular contact with the Cystic Fibrosis Unit team. It is a testimony to the vitality of the human spirit that so many mothers accommodate to these demands throughout the child's growth and development, and that so many Cystic Fibrosis patients prosper as they do, with little evidence of psychological disability.

About one quarter of the mothers suffer from depression to some degree—persistent, permeating sadness, feelings of despair, futility and hopelessness. These feelings are mostly short-term or recurrent episodes; occasionally they are chronic and require treatment.

Jobs
Among the American and Canadian families studied, nearly half of the mothers were in various jobs. In the United Kingdom and Europe the proportion was smaller: mostly, they had to give up their work and this sometimes led to repercussions on the rest of the family.

Fathers
In family groups with a Cystic Fibrosis child in which the father's reactions have been studied, the following points have emerged:

1   In over half the cases, the father appeared less concerned about the situation than his wife, and seemed to 'distance himself' from the problem.
2   In about a third, fathers did not attend the diagnostic disclosure session or the follow-up educational tutorials, and in any case appeared not to have the same grasp of the facts about Cystic Fibrosis as their wives.
3   Depression appeared much less common than in mothers.
4   About a quarter of fathers interviewed were regarded by their wives and other people as 'not pulling their weight' in home treatment and general support.
5   Many fathers felt 'left out of it'.

The Marriage: Family Cohesion
In an attempt to form a general picture of how the impact of a child with Cystic Fibrosis affects the family cohesion and

the marriage, I reviewed a number of studies made in the United Kingdom, Europe, the USA and Canada, totalling more than 300 Cystic Fibrosis families, studied for varying periods of time and by different techniques. This does not always make for measurements which some people consider 'statistically significant'; not in every case, certainly, but strong general impressions stand out.

1 In one study, Cystic Fibrosis families were compared with an equivalent group having a child with chronic asthma, and a control group of healthy families. No significant difference was found between the three groups in family cohesion and functioning, but the two groups of chronically ill children did have significantly higher frequencies of behaviour problems than had the healthy children.

2 A large group studied by Social Science academics found an increase in Cystic Fibrosis families of various emotional reactions in the parents, with marked changes in family routines—such as mothers being forced to leave their job to take care of the child, and fathers having to take an additional post in order to meet financial demands. Family reactions to the community included increased feelings of isolation, and of negative attitudes by the community towards the diseased child.

3 Group studies in the United Kingdom and Europe gave a generally more favourable picture. Most families were able to cope reasonably well with the need to adapt to the changed circumstances. Only one mother in ten was thought to suffer from depression, although many said they went through periods of dejection and discouragement. Most mothers who had been working had either to give up their jobs or cut down on working time, and some fathers felt that their increased family commitments had impaired their careers. Some mothers and some fathers complained that the adaptation process left little time for leisure activities. The Cystic Fibrosis child's brothers or sisters were found generally to be only moderately disturbed; some younger or only

slightly older siblings exhibited jealousy reactions, with rebellion, resentment, disturbed sleep and food refusal. Some felt they were neglected. Older brothers and especially sisters often showed positive and protective reactions, and acted responsibly in care-sharing activities. This was especially so when general family cohesion was good, and communication between parents and children was frank and forthcoming.

4 Two interesting reports from Sweden (where a registry of all Cystic Fibrosis patients is kept running) showed that 90 per cent of Cystic Fibrosis families were intact, and in fact in one group of 49 families studied, 19 couples felt that their mutual relationship had become better and richer for having to cope with the birth and rearing of a Cystic Fibrosis child. Thirteen couples felt the experience had changed their relationship for the worse: there were three divorces in this subgroup.

In order to look more closely at the way families respond to the situation, let us go back to James, the baby boy we met in Chapter One, and follow his progress and that of his parents, Alan and Barbara. James, you will remember, was admitted to the Regional Cystic Fibrosis Hospital Unit for detailed investigation, and the essential intensive antibiotic treatment for his early lung infection. There were usually a number of Cystic Fibrosis children there, either as in-patients or attending for regular check-ups, while their parents were learning about the treatment and discussing matters with the medical team. This naturally provided many opportunities for parents, especially mothers, to meet together and discuss their feelings and some of their worries and problems.

Emma, aged four, also an only child, had been in the unit for a week when James was admitted. She was in the next cubicle to his, her mother with her. At the time, Emma was receiving intravenous treatment through a drip into her arm and a nurse was with her, adjusting the infusion pump and telling Emma's mother that the treatment was going well. Barbara and Jane (Emma's mother) soon established a friendly rapport and liked to discuss their feelings over tea and coffee. Emma had been diagnosed as Cystic Fibrosis when she was one year old.

'We thought it all started with whooping cough three months before,' said Jane. 'My husband was against the vaccination when she was a baby. She was a lovely baby, but only five-and-a-half-pounds at birth, though she wasn't premature. I fed her myself for six months and she took her feeds well, and was eleven pounds then. I'm very glad now that I did breast feed her, because the doctors told me I gave her the best start in life; I had felt guilty when I was told Cystic Fibrosis was inherited.'

Barbara asked why Emma had to have hospital treatment with drips.

'She's got this pseudomonas germ in her lungs and has to have intravenous antibiotics from time to time, as well as the medicines I give her at home. The doctor says they can't promise absolutely to clear these germs once and for all, but they can definitely keep them in check.'

Barbara told her that James had a different germ causing infection, named staphylococcus; and that he would have antibiotic medicine continuously when he was home.

Jane said the doctors couldn't explain how Emma had picked up this particular pseudomonas germ; they said it was virtually only Cystic Fibrosis children who got lung infection with it, though sometimes it caused ear or skin infections in others. 'She gained well at first and was sixteen pounds when she was nine months. Then, when her cough started, she stopped gaining and by the time she was diagnosed she had gone down to fourteen and a half pounds. It was only then that I noticed her bowels weren't right.' Jane said Emma's motions had been normal as far as she knew, though she did tend to have her bowels open after every meal, but now they were as Barbara had noticed with James.

Alan and Derek (Emma's father) came to visit in the early evening and at the weekend, and both came as often as they could to the 'tutorials' and physiotherapy sessions. Jane had already proved a good student and helped Barbara with her practical work. The two families continued to meet after the children had returned to their homes, and the ongoing care-sharing programmes were started. Jane and Barbara visited each other frequently and were mutually helpful—Jane especially with postural drainage and effective coughing, which is not all that easy with a strong-willed little boy nearly two years old, while Barbara was expert at preparing Strawberry Milk Shake, Chocolate Coolers and other high protein, high energy drinks which Emma needed and enjoyed so much.

One day, Barbara said to Jane, 'You've been in this situation much longer than I have. Tell me, just how did you feel when you heard for the first time that Emma had Cystic Fibrosis?'

'I was shattered: I felt numb and sort of paralysed, completely helpless. I couldn't really take it in; I tried to think it would all pass with treatment and Emma would turn into a healthy, pretty girl. Derek was marvellous, he told me we would see this thing through together, but I could see he was very depressed. Then we came here, and gradually we've come to understand what it is we have to cope with; we can talk to each other about our fears and hopes. The doctor told me about my 'denial', which he said was a good defence for me just for the time being, but now I don't need it. This doctor said to me also, "Jane, you won't progress by huge leaps and bounds: it's better to make progress by little steps, which will add up to a lot in time."'

One day at the clinic, a mother who came irregularly to the follow-up sessions with her four-year-old little boy, Dean, attracted their attention. She was in her twenties, they thought, nicely turned out and presentable, but looked pale, thin and depressed. This time she came with one of the medical social workers, who went up to the doctor's desk, had a few words with him and handed in what looked like an official envelope of some kind. Sylvia (the mother) could hardly bear to let go of the child, but eventually he was let loose and joined the other children —to their great dismay. He tried to grab their toys and dolls, demolished a house carefully built from blocks by

Emma, and kicked another child on the leg. Then he burst into tears, sat himself in a corner and refused to have anything to do with anybody. He was collected by a nurse and taken, crying and squirming, to join his mother and the doctor and social worker in a nearby office.

'Well,' said Jane, who rather prided herself on her knowledge of human nature, 'there's something wrong there, for sure.'

In the doctor's office, Dean sat with his mother in a large armchair, the social worker in another, the doctor at his desk. He had read the report and had made a few brief notes to which he now referred.

'Mrs Temple,' he said, 'I'm sorry to hear things are not going well with you. Please feel free to tell me all about it. We are here to listen and advise, and to help in a practical way. There's plenty of time: I'm in no hurry.'

'Well, it's my husband you see. He doesn't seem to realise how serious it is. I don't think he bothered to try and understand. He didn't come to see the doctor after they'd done all the tests and told me Dean had the Cystic Fibrosis. He didn't want to bother with the physio or anything. I've got to do it all. First thing in the morning I give Dean the postural drainage and the slapping and the coughing. Then he gets his first antibiotic dose. After that he has his breakfast—he likes his flakes and rusks and egg—but now he wants toast and butter with honey. He drinks his milk if he loves me but he won't eat anything if I won't promise him to go somewhere he wants. They said to try him in the nursery school but I don't think I could really part with him. I know he plays me up, but there it is. The worst job is getting the enzymes into him. He takes these capsules; I can open them and sprinkle them on his food, but he loves honey so I put them in a spoonful of honey. Then, he's got to have his antibiotic medicine on an empty stomach, and his physio again in the evening, then his supper, and I've got to get his father's tea as well. I just can't cope with it all, and getting up to him at night with his cough. I feel worn out. My husband won't take any interest, he says it will all go away some day. He won't talk about it, he just shuts up

when I bring it up. He goes off to the club or somewhere.'
She hesitated; swallowed, then blurted out, 'We haven't
had SEX for months.'

Dean's father, Terry, came a short time afterwards to see
the doctor. From the social worker's report the doctor
learned that Terry was 30 years old and an electrical
engineer. He appeared reserved, on the defensive. He
asked if he could smoke.

'Not here, please,' the doctor said. 'We don't think it's
good for the patients. The reason why I asked you to come
and have a talk with me is because Dean is not getting on as
we hoped, and your wife is very worried about things in
general. She thinks you ought to take a more active part in
the treatment. What do you think? How do you feel about
him having this disease?'

'I feel left out of it,' Terry said. 'I couldn't come to the
meeting to learn all about it because of work. One doctor I
met told me Dean had six months to live, so it seemed
hopeless. I kept it to myself, didn't tell Sylvia because she
seemed to think he would get better if all the treatment was
done. I know she works hard, but it's all for him: she has no
time for me at all, and gets angry when I don't want to
talk about it. And another thing—it's upset my career. I
had the chance to go to Saudi for two years—good pay
and better prospects when I came back, but that's all off
now.'

'I know how you feel. You're not the only father to feel
left out of things in this situation, Terry. Let me tell you why
Sylvia feels and reacts as she does; also, and this is certain,
you as much as anybody can play a most important part in
getting Dean fitter physically and better able to go to school
and grow up.

'First, we know from experience now that with Cystic
Fibrosis, you can't say how long anyone's got. About 70 per
cent nowadays grow up and get jobs. It's the treatment they
get, in the family home plus visits to the unit here, which
makes all the difference. We know also, from all over
Europe and North America where Cystic Fibrosis is common, that it's in those families where both parents

co-operate in the care and treatment of the Cystic Fibrosis child, that the best results are obtained.'

Terry was now beginning to look less truculent and more interested. 'Next,' the doctor said, 'I want you to try to understand how Sylvia feels, and why. Mothers have a special relationship with their babies which we call "bonding", a joint physical and emotional link which for a time has first priority. This bonding becomes very much stronger if there's anything wrong with the child, so father for the time being has to take second place. In the case of a long term illness like Cystic Fibrosis, this bonding shows as over-protection, and father feels out of it.'

'What do you want me to do?' Terry asked.

'Actually, Terry, Sylvia needs you very much, though it may not look much like it to you, on the surface,' the doctor replied. 'What I would like you to do first is have a talk with the social worker for your case; you'll find her knowledgeable and very understanding. She'll work with you to fix suitable times for you to help Sylvia in her daily timetable. Next, I want you to learn the physiotherapy. This should be right up your street: part of it is postural drainage, and in your job you have to be familiar with pressure gradients and such like. Well, in postural drainage you use gravity plus chest pressure to help drain the bronchial tubes. It's very important, and if properly done, twice a day, it could make a big difference.'

Terry said he was interested in this, and with the physiotherapist and social worker they fixed suitable times for him to come for training, then supervision at home.

I should like now to take up some points raised in these conversations.

1 Vaccination against whooping cough is now safe and effective, using the up-to-date Pertussis Vaccine. It should not be given to children who have had a local or general reaction to a preceding dose, or have suffered from fits or convulsions. The cough of a young child with Cystic Fibrosis may closely resemble Whooping

Cough, but cough cultures would clarify the diagnosis.

2   Jane's guilt feelings when she learned about the inheritance of Cystic Fibrosis are those commonly felt by parents. We need to acknowledge and understand them; but at the same time parents can be completely reassured that they are in no way blameworthy. One person in 25 in Britain, normal and healthy in all respects, carries one Cystic Fibrosis gene. The inheritance of Cystic Fibrosis comes equally from the mother and the father. Thirdly and most importantly, having a Cystic Fibrosis baby is nothing to do with any illness, accident, treatment or anything done during the pregnancy.

3   The staphylococcus was usually the bacterium found first in Cystic Fibrosis lungs, and was thought to be the primary invader. Pseudomonas invaded the respiratory tract later as a rule, although now it does so at an earlier age and is the principal bacterium in progressive chest infection. It has proved less easy to control than the 'staph', but recent advances in antibiotic treatment show great promise. This is why Emma had to go into hospital periodically for the intravenous therapy. After a year, they hoped to lay on the home intravenous treatment for her.

4   Jane kept a reliable record of Emma's weight from birth, which was typical of a Cystic Fibrosis baby. Although full-term, Emma's birth weight was low, but she had doubled it at six months, so Jane had obviously seen to her nutritional requirements. At nine months she was sixteen pounds, again normal for her birth weight, but after the chest infection developed two things happened: first, she stopped gaining, then lost weight; second, her pancreatic function, which had been just borderline, now diminished and showed in her bowel motions.

5   Comparing Emma and James, both had Cystic Fibrosis and showed the variability of the presentation and progression of the disease, as well as the link between the pulmonary and nutritional aspects of the disorder.

6   Barbara talking with Jane, Alan talking with Derek; both
    families communicating, with spouses and with each
    other. Sylvia and Terry not communicating with one
    another, Dean showing signs of emotional disturbance.
    This is where assistance, just as much as Pancreatin, is
    needed. Communication is essential for good family
    cohesion.

The Medical Social Worker
What can the social worker do to help the family with a
child who has Cystic Fibrosis? She will have learned about
the disease generally, the various symptoms which may
occur and the treatment which is being given, and she is
aware of the secondary symptoms—emotional, psychological, and social—which may arise. Many of these can be
foreseen and prevented.

The social worker is a key member of the 'Care Givers
Network' (Figure 3). If you, the family, will welcome her,
then you will find someone with whom you can talk freely
and confidentially. She is someone who understands your
feelings, someone who can see at first hand what you have
to do in order to adapt and cope with Cystic Fibrosis. She is
also a very important liaison officer between you the family,
the Cystic Fibrosis Unit in the hospital, and the local
community. She will explain the availability of various
sources of help and social support. Some of the practical
points on which the social worker can advise are:

1   Suitable accommodation, including provision for
    physiotherapy, postural drainage and electric power for
    nebulisers.
2   Nutritional supervision and help: sometimes the extra
    food needed for Cystic Fibrosis patients requires pro-
    vision of special foods, some of which can be obtained
    on special prescription. The social worker will advise
    and liaise with the consultant and the dietician.
3   Financial assistance from Social Security. Attendance
    Allowance and possible transportation costs come into
    this category.
4   Schooling and further education.

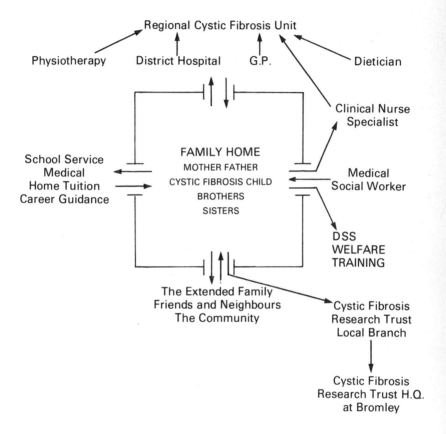

Figure 3. The Care Givers Network.

Starting School

For all five-year-old children, venturing out from the cosy sheltered environment of home to the new world of school is one of the first testing experiences of life. For parents, too, this is a somewhat anxious time. Nearly all children make the step with success and satisfaction, with maybe some temporary disturbance of sleep and eating patterns while they accommodate to the new communal life. Parents of Cystic Fibrosis children are naturally and understandably concerned about their child's ability to stand up to the increased risk of picking up infections in the school environment, and wonder whether he has the stamina for the more energy-demanding activities of the school life.

Mary, the medical social worker attached to the Cystic Fibrosis Regional Centre, knew Emma's family well and looked in to see them at home from time to time, although she knew they had no difficult coping problems now. Actually, she rated Jane, Derek and Emma as a near perfectly adjusted and adapted Cystic Fibrosis family, and often cited them to her students as exemplifying the coping Cystic Fibrosis family. 'Both parents have taken the trouble to get informed about the nature of Cystic Fibrosis, and are determined to take a full part in the comprehensive ongoing programme for Emma's health and development. We have helped them to cope with their emotions and feelings, so intensely felt at first. Derek, in spite of his work commitments, has supported his wife in every way, emotionally and in helping with all the home treatment. He has even organised things so that Jane can get some time off for herself, knowing that Emma's treatment and nutrition are being seen to.'

During one of their meetings together with other parents at the Regional Centre, Barbara and Jane were sitting with Mary.

'Could you tell us something about schooling for Cystic Fibrosis children?' Jane asked. 'I know it doesn't apply to Barbara yet, but in a few months' time Emma will be starting school, and I must confess that I'm a bit worried and uncertain about it.'

'Yes, of course,' said Mary. 'If you come in tomorrow I can have a lot of useful information for you, and we can go to see the school together, if you like. I think from what the doctors tell me there is no doubt that the ordinary school would be quite suitable for Emma. There are special schools for children with physical handicap, also the option of home tuition, but we don't think these options need be considered now.'

Next day, they met again and the social worker took Jane through the booklet *Cystic Fibrosis and You*, published by the Cystic Fibrosis Research Trust. The main points for Jane to consider were:

1 During the first year at school, all children are at some risk of picking up various infections. Cystic Fibrosis children are not unduly susceptible to this, but certain infections such as Whooping Cough, Measles and Influenza could aggravate the chest problem. Immunisation against these is available and should be reinforced if necessary.

2 Most Cystic Fibrosis children of school age have a cough of some sort, occasionally loud and loose, or 'hacking' in nature. It is important that the school staff should understand that the Cystic Fibrosis child needs to cough, and to be able to cough freely and effectively. Provision can be made for this to be arranged in the Medical Room, combined with physiotherapy. It is also important for the school staff to know that however loud the Cystic Fibrosis cough may be, the child is not infectious to other children. Some of the staff, schoolmates and their parents may be understandably worried, and need to be reassured on this point.

3 Teachers' co-operation should also be sought in arranging for the taking of pancreatic enzymes with food, perhaps also doses of antibiotics. With the approval of the School Medical Officer, these medicines could be given by a staff member, or one of the parents could be allowed to come in for a short time.

4 School meals are not the problem for Cystic Fibrosis

children that they were, now that the enlightened attitude towards plenty of normal food is becoming more widely accepted. Some parents may wish to prepare their own meals of high protein, high energy food which the Cystic Fibrosis child requires.

5 Games and PE are usually enjoyed by Cystic Fibrosis children, who do not wish to appear weaker or less active than their schoolmates if possible. When the child is well, these activities are beneficial and should be encouraged. Discreet observation is advisable, and marked shortness of breath, severe wheezing, or vomiting should indicate that too much is being attempted that day. There will be some days when activity needs to be restricted.

A few days later, Mary took Jane and Emma to visit the primary school where she was to start in a few months. Approval had been given by the Headmistress and the School Medical Officer. They were made welcome, and Emma seemed happy and quite interested in seeing what was going on, just at the end of morning break. Emma told the teacher, 'I want to come to your school. My name is Emma and I'm nearly five. I live in number 4 Claremont Gardens, with my Mummy and Daddy. I can dress myself, wash, and go to the bathroom.'

Just then, a group of children came along, formed into line and waited outside a classroom nearby.

'You see that boy, there?' said the teacher. 'That's Henry. He's a Cystic Fibrosis, and this is his second year; so now we have two.' The child she pointed out was busy swopping some small picture cards with a friend: he wasn't particularly small or thin, looked bright and active, and merely gave a 'throat-clearing' cough now and then. 'He had a rather trying time at first,' the teacher said to Jane, 'but now he's settling in very well.' Jane made a mental note to find out more about Henry, and asked the social worker if she could possibly arrange for her to meet the boy's mother.

'I don't think they come to the Regional Unit,' said Mary,

'but if you like, I'll find out and let you know. I think you'll find that Emma will enjoy school. She's an outgoing child, with a capacity for making friends and adapting. She's lucky to have such a happy home background.'

It turned out that Henry did attend the Regional Cystic Fibrosis Unit for follow-up, but because his condition had been well controlled and appeared stable at present, he did not have to attend as frequently as most patients.

It was about a month later that Jane and Barbara were introduced to Henry's mother. The nurse had earlier weighed and measured him and they were all pleased: at six-and-a-half years old he weighed 44 pounds and his height was 42 inches—a little below average for healthy boys. The doctor had told Henry's mother that his chest X-ray was clear and his last two cough cultures (taken by his GP and sent to the lab) were negative.

'How did you find out that Henry had Cystic Fibrosis?' asked Jane.

'It wasn't until he was nearly three, though we didn't think he was really as robust as his sisters, and he didn't gain like they did. He ate quite well, but his food used to go straight through him and I would see his bowel motions still in the pan after he'd been and pulled the flush. He had coughs and colds like his sisters, but the cough was more persistent.

'One day he screamed out and pulled his pants down. I saw this horrible red thing, like a growth, sticking out of his back passage. I phoned the doctor and he came straight away, took one look at it and said it was prolapse of the bowel. He got Henry to kneel down and bend over so that his bottom was sticking up; then he put on a glove, put some jelly on it, and gently put the thing back. He told me this must be looked into straight away and telephoned the consultant's office immediately.

'I took Henry next morning, and after various examinations and tests we were told the diagnosis was Cystic Fibrosis.'

Henry had stayed in the Regional Cystic Fibrosis Unit for three weeks, during which time his chest infection was treated intensively with intravenous antibiotics, and his nutrition properly organised by the dietician, with diet and pancreatic enzyme replacement. Treatment was successful: the staphylococcus was eradicated from his lungs, his bowel motions became nearly normal, and he started to gain weight. The treatment was continued at home, with antibiotic medicine, postural drainage, diet and pancreatic enzymes.

'It must have come as a great shock to you,' Jane said to Henry's mother.

'Well, it did at first,' she replied, 'especially as I didn't know what Cystic Fibrosis really was, and when the consultant and my doctor explained it to William and me, we were both very worried for a time. But, do you know, I felt a kind of relief as well, that now we knew what was the matter. I told my husband that I had been a bit worried about Henry for some time—he didn't look nearly as robust as the girls; but I hadn't wanted to worry William. He's got a very demanding job now.'

Henry's father had recently been promoted to a higher post in the Local Government Service. There were two sisters, older than Henry: Pamela aged 11 and Janet, eight.

Social worker Mary had now joined the group. She spoke to Henry's mother: 'Daphne, it's good to see Henry doing so well. Thank you for talking to Jane and Barbara, it all helps a lot when families can get together. Jane will be grateful to hear how you felt about Henry starting school.'

'Well, we were fortunate, I suppose, because William works with the Education Department and the School Health Service, so we got to know about all the arrangements they would make for Henry to have his treatment and so on,' Daphne said. 'But that wasn't what worried me. I felt I couldn't let him go into that strange new world; people said I'd spoiled him, and I suppose they were right. Over-protected and indulged him, someone said. I did let him have his own way more than the girls, certainly.'

'But what about when he actually started school?' asked Jane. 'Did he try to run home or burst into tears?'

Daphne thought for a moment. 'No,' she said, 'he

seemed to like it, and when I picked him up later, he said he loved school. But later on, his Teacher told me, he became very inattentive and often had to be told to pay more attention. She said he was quite intelligent, and when he did talk he seemed fluent and used a lot of words. He didn't like the school dinners.He said they weren't like the meals he had at home, so we arranged for him to take a packed lunch and one of the high energy chocolate drinks.'

The teacher had been very helpful, apparently, and had told Henry's mother he didn't seem over-protected. He was making friends with a few of the other boys, and played and ran about just like the others. She said he was sometimes very restless and would get up from his desk and walk around in the middle of a lesson, a rather disruptive influence, at times. On the other hand, he was very keen on school work and obviously anxious to excel. 'He could read quite well when he started here,' she remarked, and he could do sums like addition and subtraction and knew quite a few multiplication tables.'

Daphne had told her that his elder sister Pamela had taught him to read and copy words, and to do sums. 'In fact,' she told Jane, 'for a girl of her age she is very good with Henry and helps me with his postural drainage. She does breathing exercises and effective coughing with him, too, like a nurse or mother. It means I can get out a bit almost every day.'

'What about your other daughter?' Mary asked. 'Janet is not quite two years older than Henry. She's quite different and doesn't take much notice of him or play with him. I think she must be jealous that I have to spend so much time with him. She sulks and won't eat her meals if we praise him, or if anyone calls and makes a fuss of him.'

Henry's school, staff and pupils liked having him as he was friendly and cheerful and joined in all the games except the very strenuous ones. His academic progress had continued and now, in his second year, all was going well. He had had several absences when he caught a cold, as this gave him trouble with his nose and throat and his cough was temporarily aggravated, but nothing more serious had developed and he had not needed hospital treatment.

All these conversations between parents provided a valuable and therapeutic programme for understanding and sympathetic counselling. Not only the Cystic Fibrosis consultant and the paediatrician (both of whom were well aware of what was going on and highly approved of it), but all the medical team realised the important part this type of activity can play.

Jane felt much easier in her mind, and both she and Emma looked forward to the first school term after the holidays.

I should like to emphasise some of the points which emerge from these various meetings between Cystic Fibrosis parents, thanks mainly to the friendly professional help of social workers and teachers.

1   This is part of the 'Care Givers Network' (Figure 3). The best results in overall management in comprehensive care result from these activities, optimal medical treatment and the adaptive 'coping family'.

2   A number of factors help families to cope with Cystic Fibrosis: first, good family cohesion, with which goes mutual support and open discussion between father, mother, brothers and sisters; second, the ability of the parents to comprehend the nature of Cystic Fibrosis and the problems to be solved; third, the availability of local support from the DoH, the DSS, the NHS and caregivers, as well as the great help which the Cystic Fibrosis Research Trust and its local family groups can provide.

3   Operation of the recommended system of shared medical care can be seen in Henry's case, where the rectal prolapse led to immediate diagnosis and treatment, so that the chest infection was completely cleared. Henry had the staphylococcal lung infection, which is at present easier to eradicate than pseudomonas.

4   Henry's psychosocial reactions to starting school are

those reported in over one third of Cystic Fibrosis children—periods of inattention, day-dreaming, restlessness and episodes of disruptive behaviour. Between these episodes the child is happy and friendly, seeming to relish the lessening of close parental attachment and opportunities for independent functioning. Scholastic progress is usually good, intelligence normal and verbal facility usually better than average. Well before the end of his first school year the Cystic Fibrosis pupil has usually accommodated himself to the changed environment and settled in well. Truancy is actually rare.

5   The different reactions of Henry's sisters are commonly found. Sisters and brothers close in age to the Cystic Fibrosis child cannot fail to notice the extra tender loving care which has to be given to him, and are usually too young to understand what parents tell them about the special needs of the patient. So they may show jealousy and resentment, and may sulk—a sort of extension of what is termed 'sibling rivalry', seen in very many families. This is in contrast to Pamela, the 11-year-old sister, who showed a reaction often seen particularly in girls of that age and beyond: she loves to mother him, take part in giving him his treatment and adopts a caring, responsible attitude. This reflects the good family cohesion. Older boys also often display a responsible feeling for their young Cystic Fibrosis brothers or sisters, helping with postural drainage, giving medicine and going out for walks and visits.

For the Cystic Fibrosis child, the next few years at school can be happy and satisfying, provided there is reasonably good control of the lung disease and good family cohesion. The child wants to lessen the close mothering attachment which was previously necessary; he needs to develop the capacity for independent function, and feels freer and more normal in the total school environment. The concept of self-advocacy (see p. 94), which I have mentioned previously, is something that should be encouraged and supported. I know that many mothers find it difficult: 'I can't bear to let him go out on his own with his friends; I don't know what they may get up to', is a sentiment often experienced and expressed. There may be something in it, especially if normal training and discipline have been neglected. The temptation in the pre-adolescent years to keep up with your schoolmates by, say, surreptitious cigarette smoking, is an example. By this age, however, the child will have been asking questions about his illness, and he has the right to a sensible, sympathetic and truthful answer, so that he will know beyond doubt that smoking is to be avoided completely.

Susan's Story

The account which follows is based upon a real-life clinical experience covering a period of ten years. Names given to patient, parents, family and medical staff are fictitious, to preserve confidentiality; the descriptions of symptoms, investigations and treatment are true to life. Matters which have already been discussed in detail in the book are described only briefly.

Susan's story is typical of many Cystic Fibrosis children, and the importance of the experiences which I describe here in detail has only recently been appreciated. I think you should know about them, so that you will be able to deal more adequately with the problems as they arise.

The accounts of symptoms, medical examinations, X-rays and laboratory tests as well as diagnosis and treatment, are taken from the records. Various conversations and discussions described are based mainly on personal recollections and notes made at the time.

Susan was the second child of healthy parents: she seemed a healthy baby until she was six months old, when she caught a cold from her brother who was three years older. Her cough quickly got worse, she vomited her feeds, became feverish and weak. Her breathing was rapid and shallow. The family doctor diagnosed pneumonia and arranged for immediate admission to the district general hospital. Pneumonia was confirmed and Susan started on treatment with antibiotics and intravenous fluids. She improved after a few days, so that her mother, Margaret, who had been staying in the hospital with the baby, was able to go home for a few hours. When she returned later she noticed a thin plastic tube in Susan's nose. The ward sister said this was for a special test which the paediatrician had ordered, after consultation with a colleague whom he had asked for a second opinion.

Later, Margaret and her husband, Michael, had a talk with the paediatrician in his office. He told them there was something unusual about Susan's chest infection, and showed them the X-ray, pointing out the pneumonia and signs of something wrong in the bronchial tubes.

'That's not all,' he said. 'The lab grew an unusual germ from the cough culture we made. I suspected the possible cause of the infection and called in a colleague to advise on further investigations.' He paused, then said, 'Tell me, have you heard of a condition called Cystic Fibrosis?'

At that time there was less general awareness of Cystic Fibrosis than there is today, but Michael did know some relevant facts. He worked in a Government department, and a member of the staff there was Hon. Secretary of the local Cystic Fibrosis Group linked to the Cystic Fibrosis Research Trust. From time to time he put notices on the board about various events and sporting activities which were organised to provide funds for medical research into Cystic Fibrosis. Margaret and Michael had attended several of these and enjoyed themselves in a good cause. So they were not entirely taken aback, and waited for the results of the diagnostic tests.

No Regional Cystic Fibrosis Centre had been established in that area at the time, but the paediatrician's colleague was an internationally known expert on Cystic Fibrosis and only too happy and ready to assist an old friend. He was present at the next interview with Susan's parents.

'The little tube you saw in baby's nostril was to collect a small amount of digestive juice from her pancreas, for us to have tested,' he explained. 'This showed that the pancreas, although affected by the disease, is producing a proportion of the digestive enzymes, which is all to the good. The lab here did a sweat test which was positive, and I did a repeat myself which confirms the diagnosis.'

Michael told them about his contact with the local Cystic Fibrosis Group and the doctors heartily approved.

Susan improved rapidly with intravenous antibiotic treatment. The diagnosis of Cystic Fibrosis was now definite and Margaret and Michael prepared for the home care needed. They were shown the sort of physiotherapy suitable for a seven-month-old baby: postural drainage with hand pressure for the different lobes of the lungs, the baby being on her mother's knee for this, followed by coughing. Margaret was advised to carry out the physiotherapy twice daily—on an empty stomach, of course—between the 10 a.m. and 2 p.m. feeds, and again in the evening, and to give the antibiotic medicine at least half an hour before a feed. Baby Susan soon recovered her appetite and took solids twice daily, together with milk feeds totalling one pint per day. By the time she was a year old she was able to sample some of the family meals. Vitamin supplements were given daily according to prescription, also the vital pancreatic enzymes, which Susan would take as a powder with a little milk or soft food, on a teaspoon. She gained weight, so that at one year she was 20 pounds (three times her birth weight, which is normal), and her bowel motions seemed to Margaret quite as they should be. There were no chesty coughs or wheezing. Margaret attended the district hospital paediatric clinic with Susan for regular follow-up examinations, periodical chest X-rays and cough culture swabs. All was well, and the staphylococcal germs had been eradicated, although Margaret was told that it was thought wise to continue the anti-staphylococcus medicine for several years at least. Susan's weight gain continued, staying slightly below the average for her age. Her development progressed normally: at 18 months she was walking well, and could make her way slowly upstairs, holding on. She liked picture books and had a favourite doll, and delighted in pointing out correctly the doll's eyes, nose, feet and shoes. She understood a good deal of what was said and had a vocabulary of her own. Some visitors thought she was a demanding child and 'a bit spoiled', but Margaret wouldn't have that, nor did she think that she herself was over-protective.

The usual immunisations had not been given at six months, so the triple vaccine was given at 15 months, also Measles immunisation, which was recommended by the hospital.

Feeding problems began when Susan was nearly three years old. Her previously very good appetite lessened and she would not eat enough to please her parents; she would not eat the meals they thought she should have, but she wanted the things they thought she should not have. She loved potato crisps, ice-cream, chocolate, all kinds of pastry, plenty of butter on bread, cheese on toast, and anything fried. This was at the time when a restricted fat diet was considered advisable for Cystic Fibrosis children. Things her parents thought essential, such as soup, meat, fish, fruit and vegetables, were refused. Margaret's anxiety increased as persuasion, bribery and food forcing all met with defiant resistance, sulking and tears. Susan's various food fads changed from day to day, and to her parents surprise she did not lose much weight. The only untoward happening was an increase in the number of her bowel motions—up to six per day—and these were pale, greasy and very offensive. Her worried parents related all this at the Cystic Fibrosis parents' group meeting, where they learned that other families had suffered similar behaviour troubles with their toddlers. The medical social worker who was at the meeting said that food fads and rather troublesome, disobedient behaviour was not uncommon as a temporary phase among toddlers anyway.

At the next hospital check-up, Susan's lungs were pronounced free from infection, her weight was 28½ pounds, but the doctor thought her abdomen rather distended. While Margaret was telling him about the feeding troubles, Susan asked to go to the toilet and produced a typical fatty motion. The doctor did not seem unduly worried about all this. 'After the age of two years,' he said, 'children do not gain weight at the same rate as before, so their appetites are not as hearty. They are also beginning to feel just a bit independent and like to try it out on you. The Cystic Fibrosis child doesn't like to be treated differently from the rest of the family or her friends. I think in Susan's case you could be less strict over her eating habits. For one thing, when we tested her pancreas we found it wasn't totally inactivated by Cystic Fibrosis—about ten per cent of Cystic Fibrosis infants have some digestive enzymes for a time —so she could use some fat. And then, doctors are beginning to think that Cystic Fibrosis children can tolerate fat in moderate amounts, which is good for them as fat provides a lot of energy value in a diet, and research shows that they need a high energy diet as well as high protein and vitamins. So my advice would be: don't fuss, don't pile her plate full of food and stand over her. Vary the menu, offer frequent small meals of food she likes and let her have in-between snacks of high energy milk shakes, egg flips and so on. Then, a bit later, let her sit at the table with the rest of you and have small helpings of the family foods. Finally, give her more of the Pancreatin powder, not only with meals but with snacks as well, until the bowel motions come back to near normal.'

Gradually Susan's behaviour problems went away. Her general health and cheerful, active behaviour were a great relief. When she was four, she started at the little nursery school a short distance from her home. She continued with her postural drainage and breathing exercises twice daily, and with her antibiotic medicine which it was advised to continue for another year or so, until she settled in at the primary school.

Like the majority of Cystic Fibrosis children, Susan came to accept and adapt to the reality of her illness. She was fortunate in having parents and a network of caregivers with whom she could talk and discuss the 'whys and wherefores' of Cystic Fibrosis, especially what it meant for her personally. She settled in at school, made good educational progress, was well behaved and made friends easily. Games and PE she liked, and although small for her age group, she could keep up with them, apart from a tendency to wheeze with any strenuous exertion.

Her regular antibiotic medicine against the staphylococcus which had caused pneumonia when she was a baby, had been stopped after her first year in primary school. Her chest X-ray was normal and her cough swab cultures negative.

Shortly after her eighth birthday, her family and friends (and, of course, Susan herself although she didn't say so), noticed that her cough was becoming more persistent —especially first thing in the morning and after even moderate exertion. It was now regularly accompanied by wheezing. She was also easily tired.

The paediatrician's friend and colleague had by now set up a regional Cystic Fibrosis referral centre and it was there that Susan was referred. Cough swabs, chest X-rays and blood serum antibody tests showed that her lungs were now infected with the pseudomonas bacteria. She was therefore admitted for intensive treatment.

The consultant thought Susan had a right to a down-to-earth talk with him, while treatment was beginning and before her parents returned for the evening visit. 'Susan, you have done very well so far in getting on top of the Cystic Fibrosis. You have got rid of those staphylococci from your lungs; your digestion is going well with the new diet and more food intake, plus the up-dated enzymes; and you've grown and developed pretty well normally. I know your IQ is 105, so I'm sure you can take all that in.'

'Yes thank you, doctor I do understand. I've talked about it with Mum and Dad and I've read the little book from the Cystic Fibrosis Research Trust. I can do the FET (forced expiratory technique) by myself quite well now. Please tell me what's happened to me now. What are you going to do?'

'This bug you've got now, called the pseudomonas germ, has got into your lungs and it's very important to get rid of it if we can, or at any rate to keep it right down so that it won't damage your lungs for the future. We've already started with two of our best antibiotics into that drip you've got going, and after a couple of weeks you're going home to get more and better physio, plus an aerosol which I'll tell you about tomorrow and some different antibiotic medicine. Then, back to school and keep in touch with me every month. How does that sound?'

'That's fine for now, thanks, doctor, but I've got a list of questions for you. Will you be seeing me again tomorrow?'

Next morning Susan had her physiotherapy session, during which she coughed up some greenish phlegm and felt much better as the tight, wheezy feeling in her chest was now almost gone. Following this she had a lesson from the ward teacher for half an hour, including arithmetic which she enjoyed. She saw her consultant pass her cubicle with several other doctors; the group then gathered around a viewing screen studying some X-rays. They were discussing Susan's treatment. Afterwards, the lesson over and sums looked at, to be done later, the doctor came and sat at her bedside. Susan had her list ready for him.

'I know a lot about Cystic Fibrosis,' she said. 'Mummy and Daddy have told me how it makes your lungs and digestion bad, and how I've had it from birth—inherited, they said, like having blue eyes. I've got a picture book about it, written by a young girl named Anna.' Susan produced the book, which had some interesting coloured drawings as well as explanation in the text. 'But there are some questions I'd like to ask you. Why doesn't it show the pancreas in any of the pictures? My mother told me what sputum means, but does everyone have it? Can I go back to school and play like I did? Will I have to come back here again? Can I go swimming like the girl in the book?' There was a short pause, then before the doctor could begin to answer, she said, 'Will I get better? Am I going to die?'

'Susan, you're not going to die, you are much better already—I'm sure you can feel that. And you're going to get better and better as the treatment goes on. What's going to happen is this: the intravenous drip will finish in a few days, then you will have antibiotics to take between meals and I'm going to show you a special inhaler later on today and tell you how it works. The idea of this is to keep

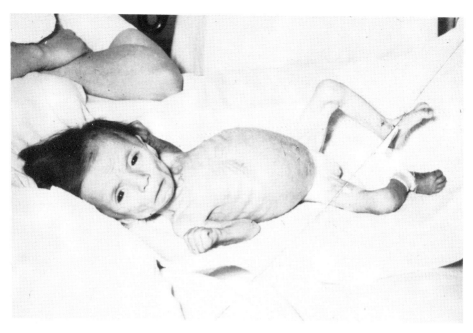

(*Above*) A Cystic Fibrosis baby in 1946 shows severe signs of general wasting and abdominal distension.

(*Below left*) A Cystic Fibrosis baby in 1984 responding well to early diagnosis and treatment.

(*Right*) Delayed diagnosis: in spite of a good appetite, this Cystic Fibrosis child has failed to thrive. His limbs are wasted and his abdomen distended.

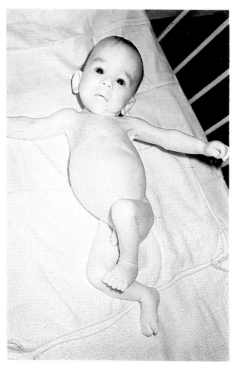

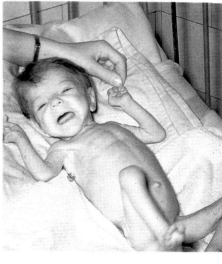

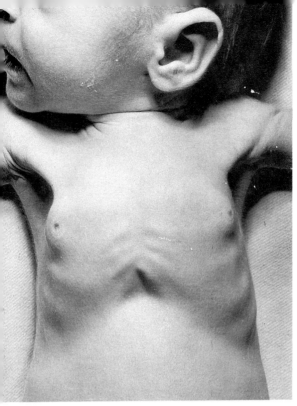

A sunken chest in a Cystic Fibrosis baby would indicate the early onset of chest infection.

An X-ray of a newborn Cystic Fibrosis baby with intestinal obstruction—meconium ileus. There is gross bowel distension with gas and condensed faecal matter producing small air bubbles in the lower left abdominal region.

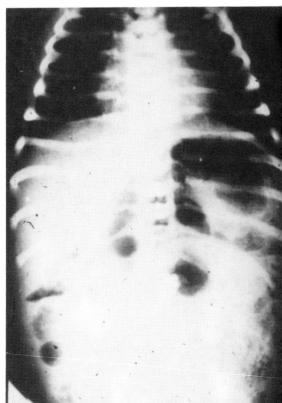

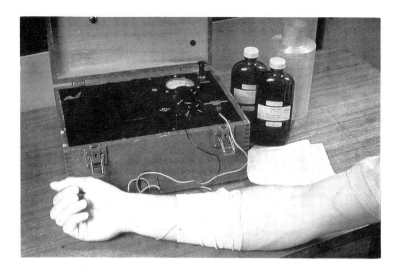

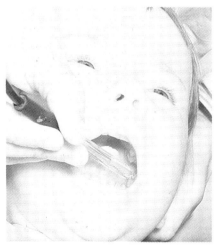

Diagnostic tests: The sweat test is still the lynchpin of diagnosis for Cystic Fibrosis. The salivary electrode test is not used much today; a new electronic potential test via the nose is being evaluated. The sweat electrode test gives a quick diagnosis but needs expert operation and is still used in some clinics.

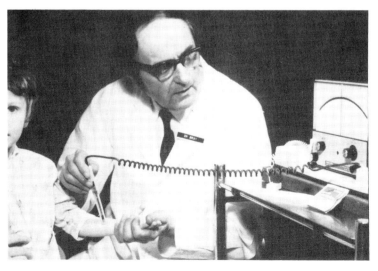

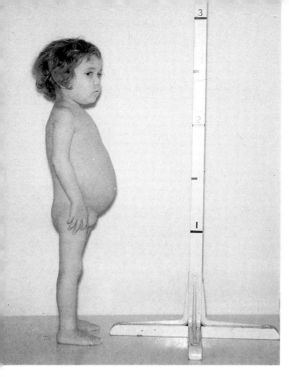

A Cystic Fibrosis toddler diagnosed at four-and-a-half years of age. Visible symptoms include abdominal distension, diarrhoea, stunted growth and a general failure to thrive.

(*Below left*) This Cystic Fibrosis teenager (1979) has been receiving the low fat diet and shows signs of general malnutrition. He has also suffered severe recurrent abdominal pains and the X-ray shows the distended bowel filled with masses of clay-like faecal matter.

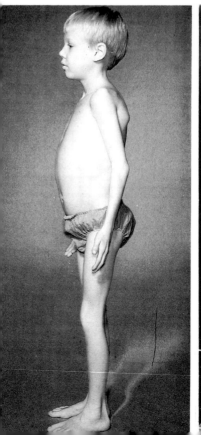

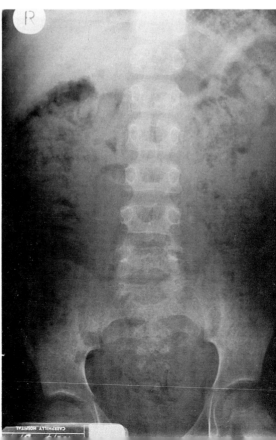

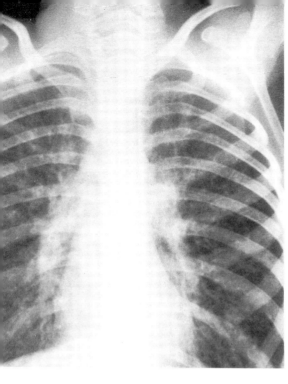

The severity of Cystic Fibrosis varies according to each patient, especially in the degree of lung involvement.

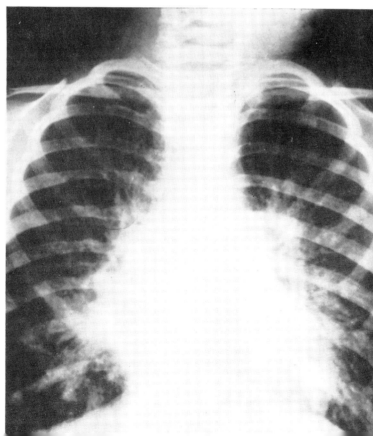

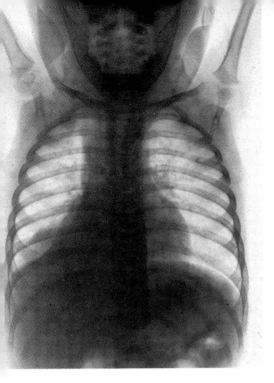 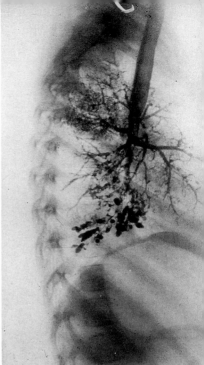

(*Above left*) The dark shadow on the lower part of the left lung is due to the collapse of the lower lobe, and when a radio-opaque fluid is introduced into the bronchus (*right*) it shows up the small abscesses which have formed (bronchiectasis).

The nose and sinuses form the upper part of the respiratory tract and their health is vital in Cystic Fibrosis. Here, the maxillary sinus on the right is filled with infected fluid and appears opaque. There are polyps in the left side of the nose.

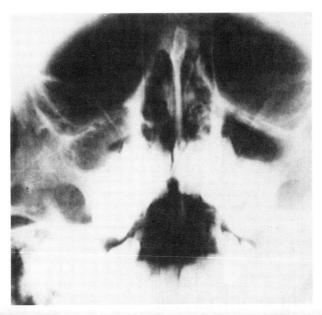

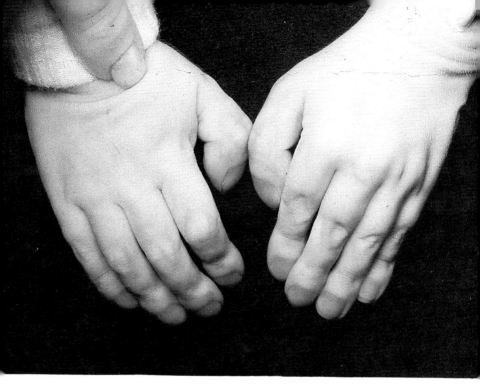

Arthritis is reported more frequently now in teenage and adult Cystic Fibrosis patients. More common than pulmonary osteoarthropathy (*above*) is 'clubbing of the fingers', associated with chronic chest infection.

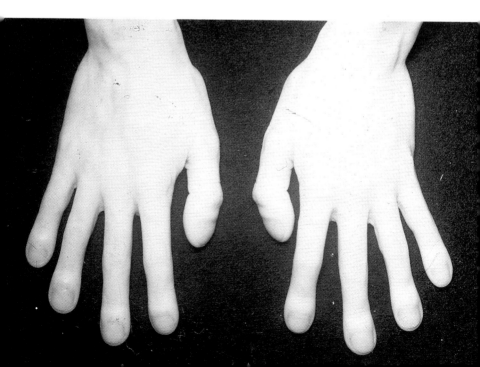

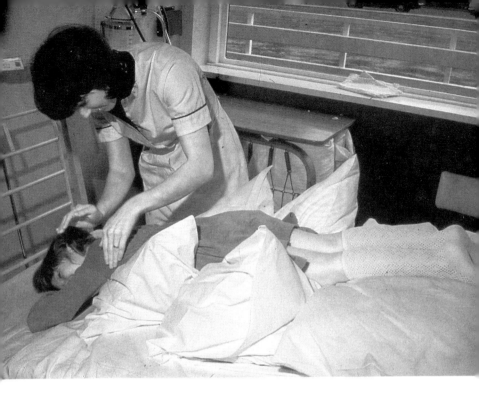

Chest physiotherapy: aims at keeping the bronchial tubes as clear as possible. It is a vital treatment, being both preventive and curative.

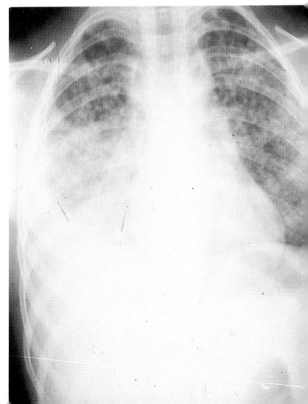

Widespread lung damage in Cystic Fibrosis can affect heart function. This chest X-ray is of an adolescent Cystic Fibrosis patient awaiting a heart/lung transplant.

antibiotics in your air tubes and lungs, also you will breathe something to loosen your sputum and open up the bronchial tubes. This part you do before your physio, and the antibiotic mist after the physio.'

When the next physiotherapy session was due, the doctor came with the physiotherapist, bringing a nebuliser worked by a compressor. This delivered a mist containing very, very small droplets of the different drugs so as to get right down into the lungs. Susan quickly got the idea, and first inhaled Salbutamol (to open up the bronchial tubes), then had her physiotherapy, followed by nebuliser again with antibiotics. She continued to improve, returned home after three weeks and restarted school the next term. She had kept up with her school work with the hospital teacher, and while waiting to return to school she had a home teacher for a month, so scholastically she had not suffered.

7 TEENAGERS: COMING TO TERMS WITH CYSTIC FIBROSIS

It is confidently estimated that by the year 1990, the number of Cystic Fibrosis patients in the United Kingdom, over the age of 13, will have risen by more than a thousand. This chapter is addressed to you, the teenagers, the adolescents, who form an important and significant group of the Cystic Fibrosis cohort.

I have enormous admiration for the way you cope with the problems of accommodating to your Cystic Fibrosis, and at the same time face up to the various tasks you have to do during this very important physiological period of life.

My purpose is to give you information about Cystic Fibrosis problems which are special to adolescence, with help and practical advice: also to provide reassurance and hope. For too long, in my opinion, there has prevailed a widespread feeling that Cystic Fibrosis is a hopeless, incurable disease—an attitude that has led to a fatalistic and passive approach to treatment and general progress.

Improved management and medical treatment over the past twenty years has resulted in much greater numbers of patients achieving adult independence in the United Kingdom and Europe, the United States and Canada. Best results are reported from specialised centres, such as the regional Cystic Fibrosis units now becoming established in different parts of this country.

Further advances along present lines in the treatment of lung infection in Cystic Fibrosis could lead to even better figures. But there is more. Progress in gene identification holds out the hope of uncovering the basic defect of Cystic Fibrosis, which could lead to the development of some radical therapy of a biological pharmacological nature.

Christine and Peter

Christine, a slight, fair-haired 14-year-old in her third year at secondary school, is doing quite well academically and taking part in most games and physical activities. The diagnosis of Cystic Fibrosis was made when she was four years old, and for the last three years her care has been shared between the family doctor, the district hospital and the Regional Cystic Fibrosis Centre.

She attends the Centre for a regular three-monthly review. There she is examined, her chest X-rayed and some lung function tests done. The physiotherapist checks on her performance of breathing exercises and postural drainage with FET (forced expiratory technique), and the dietician checks her height and weight, food intake and pancreatic and vitamin supplements.

Christine has been admitted three times in the past two years for intensive intravenous antibiotic treatment of the pseudomonas lung infection, but is now much improved. She uses a nebuliser twice daily, before and after her morning and evening physiotherapy sessions, and recently she has been taking occasional courses of the new antibiotic Ciprofloxacin, which is taken orally twice daily for 14 days.

The medical social worker, who has been an important member of the caregivers network, has recently discussed Christine's case with the school authorities, including the Careers Teacher. The Careers Service of the Local Authority has been informed and one of the Specialist Careers Officers has already had a preliminary informal talk with Christine; next year he will begin a series of 'Careers Guidance Sessions' with Christine and other teenagers who have some long-term illness involving a certain amount of disability.

Details of Christine's diagnosis and treatment have been given to the Careers Service and the Local Authority Medical Officer. Her health has improved a great deal over the past few months and she is at present regarded as 'mild to moderate' Cystic Fibrosis disability.

Let us look at the various aspects of Christine's life: the ideas she has formed about her health, what she feels about her family, the doctors and hospital staff, and the treatment she has to go through. Also her hopes and ambitions for her future career and her life-style, and what she thinks of her friends and schoolmates. She wonders what they think of her.

She is a nice-looking girl, but small and thin; her height at 4 ft 10 ins is somewhat below average for her age, but her weight, at 6 st 5 lb, is very much below average. Family life is happy, and her mother especially is less worried and depressed than she was when Christine had a severe persistent cough with vomiting, and needed several weeks at a time in hospital, three or four times a year.

Although she missed a good deal of school in her first few years at secondary level, she has made up for it by home tuition, and of course had some teaching when in hospital.

Her father, too, takes more interest in her now, helps with her school work and supervises her physiotherapy and breathing exercises. They take walks together over the hills nearby. Mostly they discuss books, films and TV, but now Christine feels she can ask some important questions.

'I'm getting better now, aren't I, Dad?'

'Yes, of course you are, much better.'

'Why am I so small? How long must I go on with all this treatment?' There was a list of further questions.

Her father had read the notes and pamphlets, and listened to some of the discussions at the Cystic Fibrosis Centre and in the local CERT Branch meetings. Some of Christine's questions were outside his knowledge and experience. He realised the importance of truthful and helpful answers, especially for teenagers. He thought further help and advice were called for.

'You *are* beginning to grow up, aren't you!' he said. 'I feel I'd better talk to someone with more experience of these things, and let you know what they think.'

Fortunately the Regional Cystic Fibrosis Centre was on the outskirts of the city. The consultant and the medical social worker were pleased to see him and thought that he had done the right thing to come to them. 'Will you let your GP know?' the doctor said. 'We'll send him a letter in a week or so. There are more and more adolescent questions coming along now, and we are thinking of organising special group meetings for them. But in the meantime, I think the best thing is for Christine to see Miss Hughes and talk things over with her. Would you like a home visit? Does Christine wish her parents to be with her, or would she prefer to come here on her own?'

Christine had no doubts. 'I think it's time I began to take charge of my own body: I'll go on my own to see the medical social worker.'

For her first session, Christine had prepared a list of questions on matters of importance to her.

'Why aren't I like the other girls? I'm small and skinny, I've no breasts, and I haven't seen my periods.'

Miss Hughes explained to her that it is very common for physical growth and sexual development to be delayed in Cystic Fibrosis teenagers, especially where there has been a good deal of chest infection. The growth spurt before puberty is delayed and menstruation begins about two years later than usual.

'Christine,' she said, 'I can assure you that your menstrual periods will come. They may be somewhat irregular to begin with but they will quickly settle down to normal.'

Christine asked about her breasts. 'They will also develop quite normally,' Miss Hughes assured her. 'First you will notice the nipples grow larger and become pigmented, and that pink circle of skin around them (called the areola) will increase in area and darken, and then the breasts will enlarge steadily.

'You'll also find,' she added, 'that your height will start to increase more quickly, and your hips will grow a bit wider, to give you a really feminine contour. Your pubic hair will grow, and some hair under your arms.'

Christine was grateful for this clear explanation and reassurance. 'I feel so relieved,' she said. 'Can I ask you about the future? Shall I be able to get married and make love? Is there any chance I could have children?'

'Of course you can get married,' said Miss Hughes. She then went on to tell Christine that pregnancy can

certainly occur in Cystic Fibrosis women, although conception is more difficult because the sticky mucus, which
characterises Cystic Fibrosis, tends to accumulate in the
neck of the uterus and form a barrier to the entry of the
sperms. A thorough medical check-up is essential.

More than a hundred Cystic Fibrosis pregnancies have
been recorded, with predominantly healthy babies, only
two having Cystic Fibrosis. Christine received this information with interest, thanked Miss Hughes and arranged to
see her again the following week.

'I feel much happier now,' she said. 'I've been feeling so
depressed at times. There are some more worries I have: I'll
think about them and tell you next time.'

As she was leaving, Christine saw a boy sitting outside
the doctor's office. This was Peter, whom she had seen
attending the Cystic Fibrosis clinics previously.

'I'm waiting to see the Senior Registrar,' he said. 'I have
my lung function tests done every month. You blow in and
out of a machine called a spirometer, and it tells how well
your lungs are working.' Christine thought Peter was a
nice-looking boy, with a refined face and nice eyes, but he
seemed small and thin like herself. 'I like the SR,' he said.
'You can talk to him about anything.'

Just then the nurse called him in for his examination.
Peter, who is 16, has needed repeated courses of intravenous antibiotics for his pseudomonas lung infection
since he was ten years old. Now he has the intravenous
treatment at home when necessary, less often than before.
Together with twice daily physiotherapy and nebuliser
treatment, he is not only in better health but much happier
and self-assured now that his hospital admissions are not
required. He does not have to miss school, and he enjoys
company and physical activities like jogging, swimming
and cricket, in which he shows some promise.

Nurse weighed and measured him. 'One hundred and
sixty centimetres—that's 5 ft 3 ins,' she said, 'and 50
kilos—just under 8 stone.' She entered it in his case notes.
He did his spirometer tests and was pleased that he did not
wheeze when he did the 'forced expiratory volume' test. At

home he did his own postural drainage physiotherapy regularly and thoroughly, plus the forced expiratory technique. The FET used to make him wheeze quite badly, so the doctor prescribed Ventolin to be used in the nebuliser before physiotherapy, and this made him feel much better.

The Senior Registrar was a friendly man of about 30, who specialised in chest diseases and had written several papers on Cystic Fibrosis in medical journals. He seemed satisfied with his examination and Peter's lung function tests. After making sure that the cough swab had gone straight to the lab, he took some blood from Peter's arm vein, 'to see if there is any sign of pseudomonas activity' and told him he was doing well. This seemed a good opportunity for a talk, as they did not seem too busy.

'What happened to George, the red haired boy, who was in the ward with me?' Peter asked. 'I see Philip from time to time—he's got a steady girl, I hear.'

When told that George (a year younger than him) had died, Peter was visibly very upset, sitting still and silent for a time. 'That's awful,' he said, 'and his chest wasn't nearly as bad as mine.' Then he pulled himself up. 'I hope to get into university in a couple of years' time,' he said. 'I'll still be able to play cricket, won't I?'

He was of course utilising the defence mechanism 'denial', which we have met before, especially in mothers. Peter was registering the facts about his state of health without acknowledging their significance, so sustaining hope and belief in his capacity to carry on and realise some of his expectations.

The Senior Registrar knew that Peter's subjective reaction was to be respected. In any case, it could well turn out to be correct, he thought, especially in view of recent advances in Cystic Fibrosis treatment.

Peter said, 'Can I talk to you about myself?' The doctor said he had about a quarter of an hour. 'Why am I so small?' Peter wanted to know. 'Not only that, but my sex development is nil. I see the others in the showers and their organs are getting like a man's and they have hair on their bellies and under their arms. I feel ashamed and embarrassed. I can see them looking at me and I'm sure they talk about me.'

'Fair enough, Peter. I know how you must feel and I'm young enough to remember how important it is at your age.' The doctor went on to say he would give Peter a very short statement of the facts, and at their next meeting Peter could tell him his reactions.

The doctor told him that in Cystic Fibrosis the physical growth and development are delayed but eventually catch up to normal or near normal. 'You see this chap here,' he said, pointing to a framed photograph on his desk, showing a young man in a track suit holding a football. 'He is one of our cases, now aged 20. He looks after himself just as you do, he's normal height and slim, and as you can see, he leads a very active life.' He looked at Peter's case notes. 'Actually, you have grown more than two inches in the past year, this is your growth spurt.'

He went on to say that boys with Cystic Fibrosis may continue to grow after the others have slowed down, and quite a proportion reach 5 feet 8 or 9 inches.

'Your sexual development will certainly become quite normal,' he said. 'Like your mates, you will find the genital organs growing larger, feeling firmer because of development and greater blood supply, and getting more pigmented. Pubic hair will grow and get curly. This is important for you to know now. There is more about future developments which I'll tell you next time. To go on with, let this sink in: we know now that growth, development and strength are related to the state of the lungs, the nutrition, and physical exercise. I know you feel that you yourself would like to be in charge of your health and vitality. That is right and proper, so think about it and tell me next time what you think *you* can do.'

He asked Peter to come to see him again the following week—not for his lungs but to continue their discussion.

Self-Advocacy: The Cystic Fibrosis Adolescent Group
During the week following Christine's visit to the Regional Cystic Fibrosis Centre and her talk with the medical social

worker, the consultant received a telephone call from the Regional Health Authority office. This was to say that an American physician who specialised in Cystic Fibrosis was over on a sabbatical to discuss recent research developments and Cystic Fibrosis management organisation, now that more and more adolescent and young adult patients were being seen. The staff were very pleased to welcome him and hoped he could stay for a time.

He arrived a week later, a man in his late twenties, rather pale and thin but otherwise well, bright and alert. They learned that he himself was Cystic Fibrosis, diagnosed in early childhood and now rated as a mild case with lung function around seventy per cent normal. His current interests during his overseas tour were genetics, the new ideas about nutrition and the treatment of chest infection, also the special problems in the care of adolescent and adult Cystic Fibrosis patients.

They had several interesting meetings. One was with the consultant, another paediatrician, a chest physician, bacteriologist, pathologist and the Senior Registrar, from the doctors' group. Also present were two of the medical social workers, the senior physiotherapist, a dietician, and a 'clinical nurse specialist'. The last member of the group was a fairly recent addition to the Centre's team—an experienced nurse who, instead of being in charge of a general medical or surgical ward, had taken an intensive course in Cystic Fibrosis and was able to cope with intravenous antibiotic drips, antibiotic doses and blood levels, nebuliser treatment and many other ward and out-patient matters, as well as home visits.

One matter which their American visitor discussed was of particular interest to the senior medical staff especially, and the paramedical people also became quite enthusiastic as the theme was developed.

The Cystic Fibrosis centre in the United States, where he worked, had set up a special Cystic Fibrosis Adolescent Group. This was intended to be quite different from the parents' groups already widely adopted in almost all countries where Cystic Fibrosis is present. The motto of the

Adolescent Group was 'Self-Advocacy', a term that I have used previously in this book.

They hoped to set up a similar group at the Centre. The aim would be to develop self-knowledge, self-care and so self-esteem, leading to independent functioning; at the same time to encourage socialisation within the group, including free discussion of problems and plans for the future. When their American guest had returned from visiting a genetics research unit they had another meeting.

He told them about the running of the Adolescent Group in his Cystic Fibrosis centre. The main features were:

1　Learning about Cystic Fibrosis.
2　Training in self-care skills, with continued support of the 'shared care' network.
3　Developing independence and feelings of control over one's health and other activities.
4　Developing the ability to socialise and to discuss Cystic Fibrosis adolescent matters with one's 'peer group' in the clinic.
5　Decision-making and the priorities in planning for the future, particularly higher education, training and career prospects.

He said that the group had been going for three years and was generally considered to be very helpful and successful. Looking back on his own adolescence 12 years ago, he wished that he could have had some of the opportunities which the Adolescent Group could now provide.

'To begin with,' he said, 'we find out how much they know about Cystic Fibrosis and its treatment, and bring them up to date. Then we organise some training in what I call self-care skills, which will make them more independent and enable them to feel more in control of their health. This is not going to be just another of those groups run by well-meaning people who tell you just what you must do. No! After the few introductory sessions, they organise the meetings and select the problems for group discussion. I know from my personal experience that we are often too embarrassed or ashamed to mention our personal problems publically, so questions and problems should be written and handed in anonymously. In our group this method gave the best results and led to full, free and frank exchanges which proved very helpful, and at the same time preserved confidentiality.'

I had met the American doctor several years before, when attending a conference in the United States. He impressed all of us with his grasp of the fundamental problem in Cystic Fibrosis, and was already making significant research progress on the scientific aspects. Naturally, the problems of adolescence were discussed. Subsequently, when attending similar meetings in America, Europe (including Poland) and of course the United Kingdom, I was especially interested to meet and discuss a variety of topics with Cystic Fibrosis teenagers in a range of cultures.

The extent of knowledge about Cystic Fibrosis, and the level of understanding and 'coping strategy', were generally good. A few places had a 'Cystic Fibrosis Girls' Group' and a 'Cystic Fibrosis Boys' Group': several had arrangements for group travel and holidays, including sports centres and ski resorts. In other places the teenagers were placed in the Cystic Fibrosis family 'chapter', together with infants and younger schoolchildren. Sometimes, at the age of 16, the Cystic Fibrosis adolescent was taken into adult medical care with patients suffering from various long-term chest illnesses, but preferably, when available, into a Hospital 'Adult Cystic Fibrosis Unit'.

Most teenagers I met in the United Kingdom had read some or all of the booklets produced by the Cystic Fibrosis Research Trust, and discussed the topics and problems described in them. A few of the older ones had 'A' levels (or their equivalent in other countries) in Biology and Chemistry, and knew quite a lot about Genetics. They all appeared motivated to be in charge of their health and life-style. A few of the older teenagers had received a copy of the *Newsletter* from the Association of Cystic Fibrosis Adults (UK).

*   *   *

I have selected some of the more interesting points which came up at meetings in various countries. Many of these I attended myself; others I learned about subsequently.

Question
Will recent progress in genetic research enable detection of heterozygote carriers of Cystic Fibrosis to be made available? Also, will accurate pre-natal diagnosis become possible? Finally, could isolation of the Cystic Fibrosis gene lead eventually to a cure for the disease?

Comments
Several members of the groups showed, from their response, that they had followed accounts of the search for the Cystic Fibrosis gene in the press (recently in *Cystic Fibrosis News*) and in a television programme. The Cystic Fibrosis gene has now been localised to Chromosome 7, and this gives hope for gene carrier detection and accurate pre-natal diagnosis.

One of the medical staff said that he had recently heard a paper given by Professor Williamson of St Mary's Hospital, London, in which he confirmed the localisation of the gene. He thought the next steps would be isolation of the Cystic Fibrosis gene and then to discover the gene product (of both the normal and the Cystic Fibrosis gene). Gene isolation would make available an accurate (99 per cent) pre-natal diagnosis at eight to twelve weeks by 'chorionic villus' sampling. The result would be available in ten days and termination of the pregnancy, if wished, at three months.

Regarding carrier detection, genetic research indicates that accurate heterozygote (carrier) detection should soon be available. There are about two-and-a-half million carriers of the Cystic Fibrosis gene in the United Kingdom, so that gene carrier detection could exclude 80 per cent of the population. The prospects of curative treatment for Cystic Fibrosis would depend upon finding the 'gene product' —that is to say, what protein synthesis the cells of the unborn baby manufacture in response to the coded message sent by the gene on Chromosome 7. Then the

long-awaited discovery of the 'basic defect' in Cystic
Fibrosis would be possible and, hopefully, remediable.

Question
The Cystic Fibrosis carriers amount to about five per cent
of fair-skinned peoples, and this relatively high gene frequency appears to be persistent in spite of the fact that
nearly all Cystic Fibrosis males are infertile, and comparatively few Cystic Fibrosis females produce children, so that
there should be a large loss of Cystic Fibrosis genes in each
generation. How do you explain this?

Comments
Understandably, there were few contributions from the
adolescents. Paul, aged 18, one of the 'biologists' (he is now
at university), had read something about this. 'Several
theories have been put forward,' he said. 'One is that there
is some biological advantage in being a Cystic Fibrosis
carrier. Inborn resistance to diseases like TB or 'Flu viruses
has been suggested, but there does not seem to be anything
in this. What they call spontaneous 'mutation' of normal
genes into Cystic Fibrosis ones is also suggested, but the
genetic experts think this is very unlikely.' So, nobody
really knows.

*   *   *

These first questions were raised by two of the older
members of the group, highly intelligent, knowledgeable
and well informed about the genetics. The comments may
sound somewhat erudite and academic, but were well
received. The next batch are quite different. After sessions
for promoting factual knowledge of Cystic Fibrosis—'What
it is', 'The genetics', 'What goes wrong in the body'—there
were discussions of the various symptoms and the treatments used. These resulted in some very interesting and
important issues raised by several teenagers, and I have
selected a few for detailed description and comment. The
first contributor was a girl, aged about 16 or 17.

What I have to put up with!
First, the treatment. Early morning nebuliser with Ventolin
so that I don't get a tight chest and wheeze when doing my
physio. This follows straight after the inhalation. First the
postural drainage with coughing, for each lung segment
followed by breathing control, then three full chest expan-
sions, breathing control again, followed by the FET—two
huffs and coughing phlegm. I don't do the slapping now.
Then the nebuliser again, with antibiotics. I make up the
solutions with saline each time myself. My mother keeps
coming in to see if I'm all right and doing it properly, she
says. Actually, I think I do it better myself than she or my
dad did it. I wish she would let me alone more.

Then breakfast and the Pancreatin capsules, which I
carry with me to school and have to take with lunch and any
milk shakes or similar. 'Look at the pill-popper!' they say.
Afterwards, PE or games; I can do most things but have to
give up if I get short of breath and cough a lot, but the
wheezing is not so bad as it was, I must admit.

Then I've got to keep up with my schoolwork. It got
behind when I had to go into hospital three or four times a
year for the IV treatment, but they helped me to catch up
and I'm going to sit 'O' levels next year.

Before my tea I have to do the nebuliser—physio—nebuliser routine again. There isn't much time for any social
life, and in any case, my mother won't let me stay out in the
evening so I miss parties and discos. I feel embarrassed
in company because I don't look attractive, I know; I'm pale
and skinny and flat-chested. Nobody tries to date me.

I get to feel really 'down' at times: can't eat or sleep, can't
take any interest in anything, feel sad and languid all the
time. Nothing seems worth while. I don't see much point in
all this treatment—in fact I forgot to do my physio and take
my capsules for three days. This may last a week or two. I
told the Social Worker: she said it was probably depression
and I ought to tell the doctor.

Comments
It was evident that this account made an impact on the
group members. Several girls had said they felt depressed

from time to time, and also felt ashamed of their bodies and the symptoms they had. Worries about the future when the time came to finish school were also mentioned.

None of the boys admitted to feeling depressed, but worry over the 'body image' was a common concern. All appeared motivated to get as physically fit as possible. One boy asked about possible use of hormones and steroids.

The natural, normal adolescent desire to break away from parental dependence is not always easy to cope with, even in healthy young people. The mood swings, the sudden changes in food habits and dress, rebellion and difficult behaviour are all familiar features of the emergent self.

Where there is a chronic illness, with varying degrees of disability, such as Cystic Fibrosis, the process of emotional de-bonding can be difficult. Adolescents with good family cohesion, with discussion of Cystic Fibrosis problems and with greater involvement of the father than was evident during infancy and early childhood, usually adjust well and come to terms with their condition. Most seem to function well on a daily level, with good academic achievement, and are able to engage in normal pursuits. The defence mechanism of 'denial' can be important to them. Cystic Fibrosis teenagers are generally good on commitment to projects, motivation, awareness and planning for the future. Studies comparing other groups of chronic handicap conditions such as Asthma, Arthritis, and kidney disease, show the Cystic Fibrosis group compares favourably, though with more anxiety about and dissatisfaction with body image, physical and sexual maturation.

Depression

This is reported in Cystic Fibrosis adolescents in America and Europe. Studies in the United Kingdom indicated a low level of chronic depression, although intermittent periods of depression, as described above, are not uncommon. These are sometimes mixed with anxiety and 'non-compliance' with treatment, diet and enzymes. Chronic depression seems more common in mothers of Cystic Fibrosis patients.

The symptoms which the family and the medical attendants would notice as indicating depression are, firstly, a change in mood to persistent dejection, unhappiness, loss of interest and general slowing up. There may be physical symptoms such as headache, fatigue, loss of appetite and disturbed sleep. Psychiatric treatment is not usually necessary.

As the patient develops a sense of control over her own health and gradually takes over her own treatment—physiotherapy, nutrition, nebuliser inhalations—with support from her family and other adolescents, so the episodes of depression will become shorter and less frequent.

Being able to discuss one's feelings, even shame and embarrassment, freely and openly with the Cystic Fibrosis group members is a great help.

Hormones and Steroids

'In the local hospital where I still attend sometimes, I've met a boy like me who wasn't growing properly or developing as he should,' said one group member, a boy of about 16. 'He said he was having injections of Growth Hormone. Would it be any good for us?'

The doctor, who was in attendance, said that the growth hormone treatment was for deficiency in the pituitary gland and would not apply to Cystic Fibrosis. 'Anyway,' he explained, 'you will have a growth spurt soon, especially if you see to your proper feeding and your chest treatment.'

Another boy said he knew of an athlete who had taken anabolic steroids, called Stromba, he thought. These tablets made him feel stronger, his muscles developed and he gained weight and strength. He knew anabolics were barred in international athletics but wondered if they had any place in Cystic Fibrosis treatment.

'I could do with some weight, especially my muscles, and maybe I would grow taller,' the questioner said. 'And the athlete said he thought his sex development had improved with the anabolics, too.'

The doctor looked thoughtful. He knew that some American Cystic Fibrosis clinics advocated anabolic steroids for selected patients showing poor growth and markedly delayed puberty, associated with digestive, nutritional and lung problems. The steroid was given in moderate to large doses for four to twelve week periods, together with intensive nebulisation therapy, physiotherapy and antibiotics. The treatment was said to stimulate growth and weight gain, the lung disease seemed better controlled and the patients reported an improved sense of well-being.

But this was when the nutritional state of Cystic Fibrosis patients was regularly quite subnormal, with inadequate total calorie intake linked with the low-fat diet then in general use, together with persistence of some degree of intestinal malabsorption and the management of pseudomonas lung infection not nearly as good as it is today. We are confident now that the new ideas regarding nutrition and the great improvement in pulmonary treatment will enable a high degree of growth catch-up, so that sexual development and maturation will be only delayed and will eventually become normal. Anabolic steroids may increase growth in height but may also stop growth earlier than would otherwise have happened, so that ultimate height is no better. Further, there are side effects of these drugs on the liver, which is affected by Cystic Fibrosis to some slight degree in many cases, with cirrhosis in five per cent of older patients.

Therefore, we do not advise the use of anabolic steroids. Similarly, male sex hormones (Androgens) are not required. Cystic Fibrosis males are nearly all infertile, it is true, but this is due to an abnormality in the tubes carrying spermatozoa from the testes (the epididymis and vas deferens) to the penis, a mechanical blockage present at birth in 97 per cent of patients. There is nothing abnormal about their sex hormones: libido and potency are normal.

There is a use for another group of steroids in selected Cystic Fibrosis cases. These are 'corticosteroids', such as hydrocortisone or prednisolone. Asthma may co-exist with Cystic Fibrosis and another allergic condition associated with the entry into the respiratory tract of the airborne fungus aspergillus, which may cause severe asthmatic symptoms—allergic aspergillosis. Both this and ordinary Asthma respond well to steroid treatment.

Occasionally, a small infant is encountered who has Cystic Fibrosis, with severe respiratory difficulties caused by bronchial congestion, swelling and blocking, with additional bronchial spasm and almost certainly infection. A good response may be obtained by adding steroids to the usual intensive intravenous and inhalation treatment.

The doctor's remarks were received with great interest and no disagreement. Before the meeting ended, one of the older girls asked to say something briefly. 'May we have a discussion with you sometime,' she said, 'about some other kinds of drugs which some of us will be meeting in the next year or two, when we go, as we hope, to university or polytechnic. I mean tobacco, alcohol, cannabis, LSD, cocaine, heroin, speed!'

Psychosocial Aspects of Nutritional Management
Until fairly recently, many Cystic Fibrosis patients, even those with some residual pancreatic function and only partial malabsorption, suffered from protein and energy malnutrition from the traditional use of a low fat diet. We have now changed our ideas and expectations for the control of nutrition, as set out in this section. As I said earlier, a poor nutritional state not only interferes with normal growth and development but may compromise the ability to resist and control infection which, for the Cystic Fibrosis child, means predominantly and most importantly, lung infection.

Present-day nutrition for the Cystic Fibrosis child means a full high energy, high protein diet with normal intake of fat and a total energy intake of 120 to 150 per cent of the normal daily recommended allowance. The dietician advises and monitors food intakes. These generous meals, which are made possible by modern micro-encapsulated pancreatic preparations, so that abdominal pain, distension and discomfort, as well as the foul bowel motions which can be so distressing and socially handicapping, should be things of the past.

Under the traditional low fat or even fat free diet, so loathed by most adolescents, the following problems arose:

1 Anorexia—loss of appetite, leading to weight loss and possible aggravation of chest infection.
2 Psychological stress because the dietary demands of Cystic Fibrosis made the young person feel conspicuously different. 'I can't eat that, not allowed.'
3 Relative isolation from friends.
4 Non-co-operation, leading to abdominal pains and abnormal, embarrassing bowel motions.

Under the new regime, temporary upsets are related to, 1) long standing dietary habits; 2) dislike or intolerance of much fatty food; 3) family eating habits, ingrained for a long time.

Questions on Nutrition

Several teenagers sent in questions about the problems they had in adjusting to the new ideas about food requirements for Cystic Fibrosis patients. Most of them had been on the traditional low fat diet at some time since the diagnosis was made. The majority, especially the boys, welcomed the change to a full diet—high energy, high protein, with a normal fat intake. A few had some difficulty in what has been called 'dietary de-bonding'; that is, the development of independence regarding food, away from mothers' ideas of what is good for you. Family dietary habits can also cause problems. In two families, what is called the NACNE Health Diet had been imposed, comprising high fibre intake, very low fat, and no sugar. This caused no trouble when low fat was the traditional prescription for Cystic Fibrosis; but now the patient and parents have to be convinced of the need for the new dietary requirement, including not only fat but the overall energy intake of 120 to 150 per cent of the usual recommended daily allowance. Cystic Fibrosis adolescents need this not only for proper physical growth, development and maturation, but to enable them to resist and control the crucial lung infection.

Employment and Training

The importance of early *careers guidance* cannot be over-emphasised. Each secondary school will have a *Careers Teacher*, who should be consulted at an early stage, say in the third year (age 14). The teacher should then (in the case of Cystic Fibrosis) inform the *Careers Service*: each branch has *Specialist Careers Officers* whose specific job is to work with young people who have some disabling long-term illness, such as Cystic Fibrosis.

By the fifth year of secondary school the Specialist Careers Officer should begin a series of careers guidance sessions with the boy or girl concerned. These will lead to some tentative choices being made, especially either staying on at school or leaving at 16 and looking for a job.

At the present time, leaving school at 16 means a choice between entering a Youth Training Scheme, facing the prospect of unemployment, or further education. The Specialist Careers Officer will be able to steer the young man or woman with Cystic Fibrosis through these difficult decisions.

In most cases there will be no need for the young Cystic Fibrosis person to be treated differently from anyone else in the scheme, although clearly environmental conditions in the workplace would be taken into account. Examples cited include the smoky atmospheres in foundries and furnaces, wood dust in workshops, some catering establishment fumes and cigarette smoke, including 'passive smoking'.

These are not, however, regarded as 'blanket bans', by which I mean that the starting point in any career-making decision should not be 'I can't do . . . this . . . that . . . etc.'

so much as what he or she *can* do, and is interested in doing.

If such choices seem reasonable to the Careers Officer and the Medical Officer, then this approach is worth trying. As I have emphasised several times previously in this book, Cystic Fibrosis care is 'whole person care', with a network of linking persons and authority: communication between the different sectors of management is essential.

The Careers Service usually deals with young people up to the age of about 21. However, as soon as anyone leaves school they may also seek help from the Job Centre. The Careers Service is run by the local Council; the Job Centre is run by the Department of Employment, and at each Centre there is based a Disablement Resettlement Officer (DRO) whose job it is to help people with disabilities to find work.

You do not have to be Registered Disabled to use the DRO, although there are some benefits in having the Green Card; as a Cystic Fibrosis person you may have an advantage, especially as an 'able-bodied' Green Card holder. Registering with the local Social Services Department as 'handicapped', may help with Local Authority grants and services. At present, my information is that less than 25 per cent of those with Cystic Fibrosis register for a Green Card. Going to the DRO has several potential advantages. The Cystic Fibrosis person who may feel somewhat unsure about the job choice can go to the Employment Rehabilitation Centre which will provide a *practical assessment* in a variety of jobs. The DRO may then be able to suggest several Government schemes which are available for people with Cystic Fibrosis, such as those aimed at helping the person with a disability to get into work—for example, the 'Job Introduction Scheme'.

Perhaps the most important part of the Job Centre service is the Disability Advisory Service (DAS), again run by the Department of Employment. Although this is primarily a service to employers, it may be particularly useful in that finance can be made available for adaptation of premises or for aids for workers with particular disabilities. An example would be the provision of extractor fans to remove fumes from working areas, of possible application for Cystic Fibrosis employees. Some Cystic Fibrosis people have also qualified for the Sheltered Placement Scheme (SPS), in which the Job Centre is also involved.

Financial Help and Allowances

Attendance Allowance
This is paid by weekly order to anyone over the age of two years (also to the mother of a Cystic Fibrosis child) who is so disabled by the disease as to require frequent attention of a physical, bodily nature, or continued supervision by day or night or both. A leaflet (NI 205) containing a claim form may be obtained from the DSS Office or through the medical social worker at the Cystic Fibrosis Hospital Clinic. The completed claim form is sent to the DSS Regional Office; then a few weeks later a doctor (Examining Medical Officer) will call to assess the patient and the home circumstances and report to the Attendance Allowance Board.

The Welfare Officer of the Cystic Fibrosis Research Trust is willing to supply a supportive letter for claimants, as it is sometimes difficult to get across the degree of intensive care and attention required for good management at home for a Cystic Fibrosis patient. The family should keep a diary showing a daily record of everything that goes on, rather like the contribution to the adolescent group meeting quoted in the previous chapter, 'What I have to put up with'—nebuliser, postural drainage, FET, nebuliser again —medication—special high protein, high energy meals and supplements, enzyme capsules; night feeds, bouts of coughing, vomiting, abdominal pain, unpleasant bowel movements at any time day or night, and so on.

Other Allowances
These may be available for mobility (e.g. transportation to hospital), suitable bedroom accommodation (e.g. for physiotherapy and nebuliser), 'whole cost' diet additions, and possibly a wider range of prescription charge exemptions.

Severe Disablement Allowance
This can be claimed from the age of 16 by those who are medically unfit for work and have been for a period of 28 weeks. If it is not claimed before the patient is 20 years old then it must be shown that he or she is 80 per cent disabled. If Attendance Allowance is being received, this counts as severe (80 per cent) disablement in the patient and qualifies for the appropriate allowance.

Income Support
Since April 1988 this benefit replaces the old Supplementary Benefit and may be claimed by those unable to work or who are out of work because of their disabling condition. Urgent payment or single payments may be met by the new Social Fund.

Students
Anyone in further education may be able to claim a special allowance, extra to their normal disability payment.

The Disability Advisory Service (DAS) and the Disablement Resettlement Officer (DRO) are valuable sources of help and advice.

The Careers Record among Young CF Adults
I have studied reports from centres in the United States, Canada, and the United Kingdom, dealing with the progress of more than 400 adolescents and young adults after leaving school.

From his famous Cystic Fibrosis Clinic in Boston, Massachusetts, the late Professor Shwachman reported the educational and careers progress of several hundred adolescent and young adult patients. Over 90 per cent graduated from High School at ages of 18–19, and two thirds of these went on to some form of higher education. Some 15 per cent received Master degrees and five per cent proceeded through graduate school, with degrees in Law, Mathematics, Biology, Psychology and Medicine. He reported that 90 per cent were 'gainfully employed', including married women as teachers, secretaries and clerks. Occupations generally included various professions, managerial positions in business, commerce, public service, industry, and tourism.

A similar series of 286 patients over 16 years of age were reported from the Brompton Hospital in London, with the great majority in either full-time education, employment or occupied as housewives, and only 12 per cent unable to work for health reasons. Another smaller group, reviewed by several of my colleagues, gave similar results. The average IQ was 105: compared with a teenage group of asthmatics, of equal ability, the Cystic Fibrosis group showed greater awareness of their ability to do something positive, even decisive, about their health. On the other hand, they showed less self-esteem and had problems with establishing their independence. The Cystic Fibrosis group were better in their commitment to vocational plans, although some of them were unrealistic in their ideas. Most of this group went on to further education or technical training, looking for careers in a profession, business management, service industry or technology.

Physical Exercise, Games and Sport
This forms an important part of the self-care aspect of Cystic Fibrosis in adolescence. Some people feel rather ashamed of their relatively poor physique, and dislike undressing in front of their friends. Others notice that exertion may bring on a bout of coughing, sometimes with wheezing. Most enjoy some form of physical activity and feel better for persevering.

The medical reasons for recommending physical exercise are:

1   Attaining a degree of fitness off your own bat increases the feeling of control over one's health.
2   It has been shown by scientific measurements that regular exercise and games, tailored to your individual capabilities, increase the efficiency of the lungs, heart, and circulation.

3   For boys especially, but important also for girls, the
    general physique is improved, and certain exercises
    help in muscle growth and power in legs, arms and
    shoulders. The important respiratory muscles take part
    in this improved strength.

These activities should complement your regular
physiotherapy, not replace it, however tempting that may
be. A practical compromise could be to do one daily physiotherapy session, say in the early morning, and one
equivalent exercise or games session later in the day. The
important thing is regularity: *something* must be done *twice*
each day. If you intend beginning this kind of 'positive
health promotion', this is how to set about it.

First, consult the doctor you usually see at the Cystic
Fibrosis Clinic and tell him what you have in mind. He or
she will go over your medical file, examine you and check
your lung function tests. What is called an 'Exercise Toler-
ance Test' will probably follow. This consists of a standard
set of exercises, with running, use of a cycling machine and
possibly other exertion for a period suited to your state of
health. At the end of this you will probably feel short of
breath, which is normal; your heart rate, respiratory function and perhaps blood pressure will be checked, then
measured again at one minute, two minutes, and maybe
later if necessary.

The doctor will then be able to advise you about your
future plans, the degree of competitive sport you may be
able to attempt eventually, and how to begin and, hopefully, to progress. To start with, perhaps just regular daily
walks, or a cycling or rowing machine; then gentle jogging,
running, tennis, badminton, swimming (better not diving,
to start with, anyway), leading, if all goes well, to football,
hockey, cricket or baseball.

Exercise naturally makes one short of breath sometimes,
but this quickly settles down. If the breathlessness persists
and you feel exhausted, this means you have overdone
things for the time being and should go back a stage.
Coughing and sputum production are nothing to worry

about: after all, this is the aim of much physiotherapy. Wheezing, however, especially if regularly occurring or persistent, is a different matter.

Wheezing may occur in Cystic Fibrosis patients for three reasons:

1 What is termed *'bronchial lability'*, peculiar to the disease and believed to be due to a combination of viscid mucus accumulation, swelling of the bronchial walls and probably some infection, plus bronchial spasm. It occurs in the smaller airways and usually shows itself early in the course of the disease, often in infancy where it may prove distressing. It is possible but unlikely to occur for the first time in adolescence.

2 *'Allergic aspergillosis'*, a fungal infection affecting the respiratory tract, due to bronchial spasm secondary to the infection; this again is unlikely to show itself for the first time in an adolescent taking exercise. The chest X-ray and a specific blood test will make the diagnosis.

3 *Asthma* is common (about three per cent of all school-children), less so in adolescence, and may easily co-exist with Cystic Fibrosis. There is a strong hereditary predisposition, with family history of asthma, wheezy bronchitis or hay fever, and infantile eczema. Exercise-induced Asthma may occur in susceptible adolescents, especially in cold, windy weather. Vigorous physiotherapy may occasionally bring on wheezing in patients with hereditary tendency to asthma, and Salbutamol aerosol is a useful preventative measure in this and exercise-induced bronchospasm—for example, one to two puffs of Ventolin inhaler before physiotherapy or physical exertion.

A number of adolescent and young adult patients known to the Cystic Fibrosis Research Trust are able to take part in competitive athletics, football, tennis, cycle racing, swimming galas, golf tournaments and other testing physical activities, without harm but with positive well-being, including heightened self-esteem and realistic future planning.

Salt Depletion, Heat Prostration, Heat Exhaustion
These are different names for the same condition, usually produced by exposure to heat, especially in hot, humid weather, by people not acclimatised to such conditions. There is excessive sweating, leading to loss of salt (sodium chloride) and water. It is easy to see how Cystic Fibrosis patients with a five-fold sweat salt content may fall victim to this illness, especially enthusiastic young people embarking on strenuous physical exercise.

The symptoms are weakness, cramps, vomiting and collapse, with very low blood pressure. Treatment is by intravenous glucose-saline solution. Prevention (obviously better!) is by avoiding such exposure, by drinking salt and glucose solution before exercise in very hot weather, or by taking, for example, enteric-coated 'Slow Na' tablets.

Physical Symptoms in Adolescence
Certain symptoms may be encountered for the first time during adolescence, in a known Cystic Fibrosis patient. Occasionally, one of these symptoms may occur in a teenager or even young adult who has not been previously diagnosed as having Cystic Fibrosis, signalling the need for diagnostic tests. Diagnosis may be difficult in some adolescent or adult cases, because the sweat test is not as decisive as in infancy and childhood. There are, however, special modifications of the sweat test, which, together with pancreatic function tests and chest X-rays, will enable a firm diagnosis of Cystic Fibrosis to be made. It is possible that there exists a relatively mild type of Cystic Fibrosis, in which the patient retains some pancreatic enzyme function for a long time and suffers a lesser severity of chest infections.

Abdominal pain is common in Cystic Fibrosis patients of all ages, usually colicky in type, intermittent and accompanied often by flatulence and abnormal bowel motions. These symptoms usually pass off after a day or two, but should always be reported to your doctor. Severe persistent abdominal pain, especially when felt in the right lower quarter of the abdomen, is a more serious matter and needs urgent investigation and treatment. There is usually constipation, loss of appetite, and sometimes vomiting also. The abdomen becomes swollen and the doctor will probably feel a smooth, mobile, indentable, and usually non-tender lump in the right lower abdomen. This condition, when first described, was termed 'meconium ileus equivalent' because there is an accumulation of firm, undigested material including precipitated protein and fat, mixed with coagulated muco-protein in the last portion of the small intestine. This was thought to resemble the meconium ileus obstruction encountered in ten to fifteen per cent of newborn Cystic Fibrosis babies, but there is no real connection between the two conditions. You may read or hear the term 'DIOS' used to denote this symptom: it stands for 'distal intestinal obstruction syndrome', which is treated now by special enemas (Airbron or Gastrografin), tube feeding and intravenous fluids. Today surgery is rarely necessary. After recovery from an acute attack, there is a careful review of the patient's dietary habits and especially the type, dose and practical administration of the pancreatic enzymes, because faults in one or more aspects of these may underlie the symptoms. The new enteric coated microspheres (Creon or Pancrease) should be given in suitably large doses to cope with dietary intake, and perhaps aided by Cimetidine or Ranitidine to reduce the stomach acid output. Several members of one group I met related their experiences of DIOS, which in two cases had occurred off and on since early childhood, and in another had led to operation for suspected appendix abscess.

Doctors must of course consider other causes of abdominal pain when making the diagnosis, including appendicitis, intussusception, even such things as peptic ulcer, gallstones and inflammation of the pancreas (pancreatitis) which may occasionally occur in Cystic Fibrosis (see Figure 4).

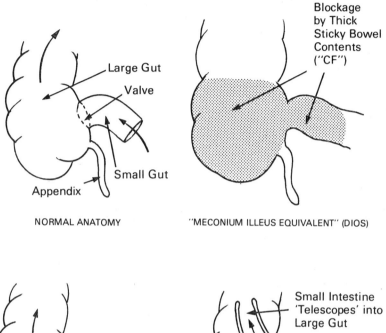

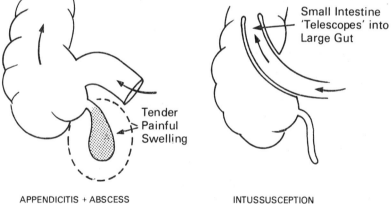

Figure 4. Mechanisms of abdominal pain in Cystic Fibrosis.

An older girl once asked me about *Diabetes*. She had met a young man of 22 on holiday, and since then they had exchanged letters about once a week. He had told her that he had Cystic Fibrosis and attended one of the regional Cystic Fibrosis referral centres in the north of England. In his last letter he had said he had been losing weight recently and felt very thirsty, even during the night; the consultant had carried out some urine and blood tests and told him he had a mild form of Diabetes, which could occur in one in ten Cystic Fibrosis people of his age group and older.

The diabetic tendency may be found during a routine visit to the Cystic Fibrosis Centre, in a patient who has none of the classic symptoms. The urine test shows that glucose is present (glycosuria) and a simple blood test shows an abnormally high glucose level (hyperglycaemia). About one quarter of Cystic Fibrosis schoolchildren and adolescents show glucose intolerance when given a test dose, and one large group studied revealed about 12 per cent with mild diabetes. As a rule this shows as a loss of weight, marked thirst and greatly increased fluid intake and urine output. The condition is usually easily controlled by diet and drugs such as Rastinon, which help to control the blood sugar; about one third of Cystic Fibrosis diabetics require small doses of insulin to control the condition. The unpleasant long term complications seen in some non-Cystic Fibrosis patients have not so far been reported in our group.

We (patients and doctors) quite rightly attach major importance to the chest in the overall management of Cystic Fibrosis, concentrating on the bronchial tubes and the lung segments with antibiotics taken intravenously, orally and by inhalation, and with the essential physiotherapy, breathing exercises and physical training.

Sometimes, in our enthusiasm for this prime objective, we are apt to overlook that part of the respiratory tract which begins at the nose, then continues through the sinuses and the back of the throat (naso-pharynx) down to the trachea.

During one meeting, when wheezing in Cystic Fibrosis teenagers during physiotherapy and physical exercise was

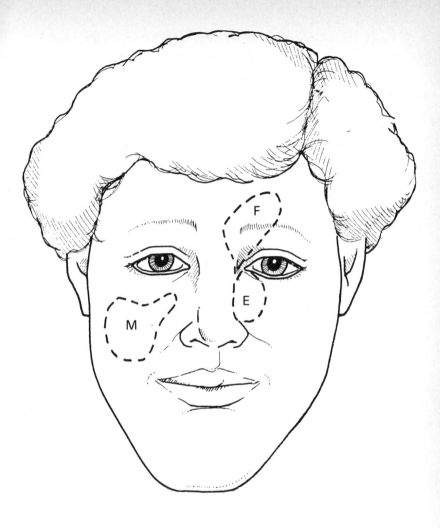

Figure 5. The upper respiratory tract. The nose and the sinuses are essential parts of the respiratory tract, and are often involved in Cystic Fibrosis. The figure shows the sites of pain and tenderness where the sinuses (which are bilateral) are affected.

F = frontal sinus. E = ethmoidal sinus. M = maxillary sinus (often filled with mucus and pus). Nasal polyps grow from the sinus openings.

being discussed, a sixteen-year-old named Debbie asked, 'Is *Hay Fever* a part of Cystic Fibrosis? I know you told us that Asthma and Bronchial Spasm can occur, and my cousin who is not Cystic Fibrosis has Asthma, and gets Hay Fever each spring. I don't wheeze, but lately, although it's winter, I've been sneezing a lot and my nose is often blocked up or discharged. And I get pains just around and over my left eye.'

The doctor said he thought the symptoms could well be caused by sinusitis, and arranged to examine Debbie after the meeting. He found tenderness on pressure over the frontal and ethmoidal sinuses (see Figure 5, areas F and E) on the left side. An X-ray confirmed sinusitis and indicated the presence of nasal polyps. Debbie said she had recently had a rather heavy cold and admitted that when she went to the swimming pool she sometimes dived in feet first from a height.

The nasal cavities and the sinuses are lined by a mucous membrane resembling that of the lower respiratory tract, so that sinusitis of some degree is common in Cystic Fibrosis. The situation can be aggravated by Allergic Rhinitis (Hay Fever) which occurs in Cystic Fibrosis as much as in people generally. Severe acute sinusitis, requiring repeated drainage operations, is very rare in Cystic Fibrosis, but nasal polyps are reported as occurring in ten per cent of adolescent and 25 per cent of adult Cystic Fibrosis patients. Treatment for polyps is, firstly, a nasal spray such as Beconase, which will relieve congestion and nasal obstruction, and secondly, an operation to remove the polyps. These benign polyps may, however, grow again and further surgery may be required to relieve the obstruction and complete the removal of the polyps. The underlying cause of the problem is sometimes allergic.

Another teenager brought up the question of *Arthritis* in Cystic Fibrosis. She said she knew a woman, not with Cystic Fibrosis but with chronic bronchial disease, who had painful swellings of the knees and ankles lasting a long time. This patient had been investigated in hospital and her X-rays had shown abnormality in some of her bones. The questioner said that she herself had recently suffered from pain and swelling in her knees and left wrist. Her doctor had diagnosed polyarthritis and prescribed Brufen tablets, and the symptoms had cleared up before her next visit to the clinic three weeks later. Someone else in the group knew of a Cystic Fibrosis teenager who had suffered several attacks of pain and swelling in the joints, so that Rheumatoid Arthritis had been suspected. The symptoms came and went over a period of several months and then ceased.

The subject of Arthritis and Cystic Fibrosis has fairly recently been studied, now that there are many more adolescents and adults in the total Cystic Fibrosis population, as it is that age group which is affected by joint problems. The first type, which occurs with long-standing lung disease combined with infection, has a long name of Greek and Latin origin—Hypertrophic Pulmonary Osteoarthropathy—which means literally 'suffering with joints, and bony overgrowths, to do with the lungs'. This condition has been known for a long time in patients with chronic chest disease. The larger joints, knees and ankles are mostly affected, but also the hands, where there is swelling of the bones between the finger joints. Now that the prevention and treatment of tuberculosis, bronchial and pulmonary abscesses and empyema are so much more successful, osteoarthropathy has become much less common. Cases have been described in Cystic Fibrosis adults, but in my experience it is unusual. There is a striking difference between the hands in pulmonary osteoarthropathy and the much commoner 'clubbing of the fingers' in Cystic Fibrosis, due to overgrowth of soft tissues at the bases of fingernails and toenails, which is also associated with chronic chest infection.

Rheumatoid Arthritis is a slowly progressive, intermittently occurring, generalised disease, mainly of adults. It affects the joints, especially those of hands and feet, together with other symptoms such as fever, loss of weight, rapid heart action, nodules under the skin and often a fleeting, recurrent rash. It affects girls twice as often as boys, sometimes early in life between two and five years old

(Still's Disease) and again in adolescence and early adult life. The diagnosis is made from the symptoms plus specific laboratory tests. It may therefore occur in Cystic Fibrosis patients, but again, like pulmonary osteoarthropathy, it is in my experience uncommon.

Other causes of painful joints which have been reported in Cystic Fibrosis are inflammation of the pancreas (Pancreatitis) and excess uric acid in the blood: both are rare. German Measles (Rubella) is frequently acompanied or followed by joint pains, but here, of course, the diagnosis should be obvious.

What is now receiving increasing attention is the condition termed 'Cystic Fibrosis Arthropathy', which is reported as occurring in about eight per cent of adolescent and adult Cystic Fibrosis patients. Symptoms are pains in some joints, most often the knees, which are worse after standing about; the wrists may also be affected The joints feel warm to the touch, and the doctor may find signs of fluid (synovitis). The symptoms usually subside gradually with or without treatment, although the knees usually need rest. After a week or so, pain and swelling have gone. In some cases the symptoms have come back, then remitted, only to return once or twice over a period of six to nine months before finally ceasing completely. In one patient, the wrist pain and swelling involved the tendon sheaths as well as the joint (teno-synovitis). No constitutional or general organ involvement has been seen in these cases, but in a few the blood serum showed a positive result for 'rheumatoid factor'. This finding by no means indicates any definite sign of Rheumatoid Arthritis, as it has been found in many cases of chronic lung infection, including Cystic Fibrosis.

One possibly important finding recently reported from Cystic Fibrosis units at the University Hospital of Wales and the Brompton Hospital, is the apparent association of Cystic Fibrosis Arthropathy with the oral antibiotic Ciprofloxacin, which is a recently introduced effective drug against the Pseudomonas and a valued addition to the overall treatment of Cystic Fibrosis lung infections. Too much need not be made of this, but it would be wise for patients and doctors to be aware of the association and report any joint symptoms. After all, cases of Cystic Fibrosis Arthropathy were known before Ciprofloxacin was in use. Dr Goodchild states that the manufacturers of Ciprofloxacin reported cases of joint pains (knees and ankles) in two Cystic Fibrosis girls, out of 49 Cystic Fibrosis patients receiving the antibiotic. Any previous possible side effects to antibiotics, for example, urticarial rashes, gastro-intestinal upsets and occasionally joint pains, should be reported when treatment with a new antibiotic is suggested.

Smoking, Drinking and Drugs

One topic for discussion and advice at our meetings was the effects of Cystic Fibrosis on the patient's liver. A question regarding this was put by a seventeen-year-old boy. 'My uncle died recently,' he told us. 'He was only 50 years old. My father said it was cirrhosis of the liver caused by heavy drinking for a long time. I drink once or twice practically every week, about five pints of beer a week, I suppose —sometimes wine or cider, never spirits. I read in the Cystic Fibrosis Research Trust booklet called *Cystic Fibrosis and You* that some people with Cystic Firosis have problems with their liver. Could I get cirrhosis of the liver? Should I give up drinking altogether?'

I was intrigued to learn from the discussion that nearly all in the group had taken some alcoholic drink at one time or another; many had had a drink within the last week, and some said they drank regularly every week, girls as much as boys.

The general subject of smoking, drinking and drugs seemed so important that they decided to devote a whole session to it. Julie (17 years) said she would collect some general impressions and possibly some experiences from her group of Cystic Fibrosis friends.

Before the meeting, I made some notes giving the results of several surveys carried out by health and educational authorities between 1985–87, relevant to attitudes towards health and medical problems in teenagers. More than

25,000 adolescents in areas including London, the Oxford area, Devon and Wales, answered questions dealing with a great range of health matters. The age range was between 14 and 18 years, the majority being 16 to 17.

Smoking

Thirty-eight per cent of boys and 33 per cent of girls said they had never smoked, while 27 per cent of boys and 24 per cent of girls said they had smoked 'just once or twice'. One quarter of the 16 to 17-year-old boys and one third of the girls admitted to being regular smokers; seven per cent said they smoked between six and nine cigarettes a day on average, two-and-a-half per cent said ten to fifteen a day.

Between 70 and 98 per cent in the different groups, more so among the 14–15-year-olds, said they thought 'smoking could damage your health'; only seven to ten per cent thought 'there is nothing wrong with smoking'.

All these teenagers were regarded as generally healthy: two per cent suffered from Asthma, and two per cent had weight problems, joint pains or frequent colds. There was no figure given for any Cystic Fibrosis patients.

Drinking

As many as 95 per cent said they had taken an alcoholic drink at some time. Of the 16–17-year-old group, more than half had taken one or more drinks during the previous week, and 32 per cent were regular weekly drinkers. Eight per cent of boys and 14 per cent of girls said they merely had one beer or one glass of wine per week; at the other end of the scale, seven per cent of boys and three per cent of girls (16–18 years old) said they consumed ten pints of beer or 20 glasses of wine per week.

Drugs

The overall incidence of 'solvent' or 'glue' sniffing was five per cent, relatively higher in the 14–15 age group; other drugs, not specified, had been tried by nine per cent in the total age range. There appeared to be an association between smoking, drinking and drug taking.

So much for the attitudes to health and living styles of a large representative sample of teenagers from the southern part of the United Kingdom. Fashions change in these matters during adolescence, as they do regarding foods, dress, hair styles and behaviour patterns. The emergent self feels the need to look into and perhaps test all aspects of social living. Pressures come from all sides: from authority figures, from peer groups, and from idealism and emulation of popular heroes and heroines in music, acting, fashions, athletics and games.

*   *   *

When we come to Cystic Fibrosis adolescents, there are some facts we should study regarding smoking, drinking and drugs. There may be a kind of 'group opinion' as to what attitude Cystic Fibrosis teenagers should take about these matters, but individuals will make up their own minds. Apart from smoking, I am not going to browbeat anyone to try to make your flesh creep.

Smoking and Cystic Fibrosis
Cigarette smoking is, in my opinion, a repellent, dirty and anti-social habit which has been shown decisively to lead to lung diseases such as bronchitis, emphysema and cancer, and to coronary heart disease. This view has become increasingly supported by all groups of society over the past twenty years. The health of the respiratory tract from the nose to the base of the lungs has been shown to be the most important single factor affecting the quality of life for Cystic Fibrosis people. There is more. Not only does active cigarette smoking have harmful effects on your own bronchial tubes and lungs (and eventually, your heart) with all the side effects on physical fitness and general well-being, but 'passive smoking' has recently come to the fore as a sinister ally of the cigarette.

'Active smoking' includes lighting the cigarette, placing it between the lips and inhaling the smoke through the filter tip into the mouth or deeper into the air passages, followed by exhaling or blowing the smoke out into the surrounding air, where it disperses. This air is inhaled by other people, constituting passive smoking. Some smoke comes from the far end of the cigarette, whether it is in the mouth, held in the fingers or left burning in the ash tray. This smoke has never passed through the filter, but it disseminates just the same into the air which someone else is going to inhale. This is also passive smoking. Recent experiments showed a definite toxic content of smoking products in the atmosphere round about.

Cystic Fibrosis people should therefore never smoke. In the family home, communal lodging, places of study, training or work, it is obviously desirable that passive smoking should be controlled by setting aside certain ventilated rooms for smokers. Places of entertainment and enjoyment should also be made as free from toxic tobacco products as possible. I know this is not easy at present. A forthcoming Department of Health publication deals with this problem and makes important reading for all of us.

Like some other things which are potentially very bad for you, cigarette smoking may acquire a certain shady glamour. Part of the adolescent process of achievement of independence of thought and behaviour is rebellion against authority, breaking the rules and trying anything.

When we began our meeting on this whole subject, Julie told us about an article she had read in a national newspaper on the subject of a new fashion-world publication. It featured a double-page spread showing forty famous and glamorous people, and with a pointing finger said, 'Do these people *still* smoke?' Some people apparently think 'all terribly glamorous women still smoke'.

The writer had the same feelings about smoking as those I have described above, and emphasised the increased risk of lung cancer and coronary heart disease for women who now smoke regularly. She described a very elegant fashion, model, photographed on the Chanel cat-walk in Paris with a cigarette in her hand, in defiance of the opinion that cigarettes and glamorous people should not be seen together in public places.

Julie had taken a confidential census of smoking habits among the 11 Cystic Fibrosis teenagers of her acquaintance. None were currently smoking, nor had any of them smoked at all within the past three years. Two said they had tried 'the odd cigarette' on occasion, 'just to see what it was like', but had quickly realised it was a bad habit.

The group opinion was unanimous: smoking for Cystic Fibrosis people is utterly disastrous; they themselves would never smoke, and they would do their utmost to convince any Cystic Fibrosis child with whom they came in contact that smoking was out as far as they were concerned. Not only that, but most thought more should be done to minimise passive smoking, especially in places of work, residence and leisure, and at all indoor public functions.

Drinking

We raised again the matter of the boy's uncle who had died at the age of 50 from cirrhosis of the liver, brought on by heavy drinking over a long period. The Cystic Fibrosis Research Trust booklet mentioned by the boy includes the question, 'Can I drink *any* alcohol?' and the reply is, 'This will depend on how well your liver is functioning. Some people with Cystic Fibrosis have problems with their livers. It could also depend on what medicines you are taking. The best advice would come from your doctor.'

Opinions on this subject were not so uniform as with smoking. Some felt that 'controlled drinking' could be acceptable, keeping to the guidelines indicated by the Royal College of Physicians—so many 'units' of alcohol per week, for example. They knew of a number of people in Britain and Europe who had drunk moderately from youth to a ripe old age, with no symptoms of liver disease. One said he had read of liver cirrhosis occurring in teetotallers (even children) in India. Several people pointed out that at the regular check-up at the regional Cystic Fibrosis centre, the liver and spleen were always examined by Ultra-Sound, and blood tests for liver function were regularly done, so that at the first sign of any liver trouble one could abstain completely.

The medical facts concerning the liver and Cystic Fibrosis are as follows:

1 *Some* slight evidence of liver involvement can be found in most cases of Cystic Fibrosis, even in newborn babies (some have prolonged jaundice). Microscopical examination shows the small bile channels plugged with viscid bile in various focal areas which are accompanied by proliferation of the ducts and some fibrous tissue round about, in scattered sites. Professor Bodian described this 'focal biliary fibrosis' as typical of Cystic Fibrosis. It is, of course, quite different from alcoholic cirrhosis, and in the great majority of patients never progresses to that serious condition.

2 In about a third of Cystic Fibrosis children the liver shows an abnormal deposition of fat, probably connected with dietary deficiencies. This does not lead to any serious symptoms, and with modern diet, vitamin supplements and effective pancreatic enzyme treatment, should become less common.

3 Long-term follow-up examinations have shown that about five per cent of adults with Cystic Fibrosis have true 'multilobular' cirrhosis of the liver. It is not known why the early changes mentioned above should progress in such a small proportion, or why an even smaller number—under two per cent—have the serious liver problems (portal hypertension) which afflict the alcohol-related type of liver cirrhosis.

It seems possible that Cystic Fibrosis liver disease in adults could be partly the result of nutritional problems earlier in life, plus the small bile-duct fibrosis. If so, modern nutritional dietary treatment should result in some improvement. As regards alcohol, I agree with the Cystic Fibrosis Research Trust booklet: consult your Cystic Fibrosis clinic.

Drugs and Cystic Fibrosis

CANNABIS is the botanical name for the genus of hemp plants (*Cannabis ativa* or common hemp; *Cannabis indica* or

Indian hemp); it is also the name of the narcotic drug obtained from the resin and from the dried leaves and flowers. The drug cannabis is also known in various parts of the world as hashish, bhang, marihuana, etc. It is taken by smoking, either as a cigarette or in a kind of pipe. It acts as both depressant and stimulant of the central nervous system, claimed to give a state of relaxed well-being. Side effects are reported as impaired short-term memory and concentration, sometimes feelings of unreality and depersonalisation. Cystic Fibrosis people should note that increased heart rate, raised blood pressure, and bronchitis are also seen in smokers of 'pot'.

AMPHETAMINES include dexedrine, durophet and similar drugs which were formerly used medicinally in the treatment of obesity and some forms of depression. Because of their liability to become addictive and their toxic effects —hallucinations, delirium, rapid and irregular heart action and raised blood pressure—their use is now limited to a few specific conditions, and they have no place in the treatment of obesity. They tend to retard physical growth, and the anorexia which they induce would lead to undesirable weight loss in Cystic Fibrosis patients, with possible impairment of the body's ability to resist lung infections.

BARBITURATES, including such well-known names as Amytal, Nembutal, Seconal, were formerly prescribed by doctors for a variety of nervous disorders, but their tendency to cause drug dependence, combined with such toxic side effects as respiratory depression, has produced a marked decline in their use.

BENZODIAZAPINES have largely taken the place of barbiturates for the treatment of insomnia, anxiety states and various other nervous disorders. Diazepam (Valium) is a well-known and often prescribed drug for anxiety symptoms, while nitrazepam (Mogadon) and temazepam are commonly used for sleep disorders. The benzodiazepam drugs have less frequent side effects than barbiturates and are generally less dangerous in overdosage but occasionally produce unexpected outbursts of hostility and aggression, especially in conjunction with alcohol. Some drugs in this group also have a hangover effect, which may slow down reactions and judgement and so affect the ability to drive or operate machinery. This effect occurs particularly with regular nightly doses which gradually accumulate, and is increased by alcohol consumption. Dependence is not uncommon, and Cystic Fibrosis people should note that in chronic respiratory disease doctors are advised to use caution in prescribing any of this group of drugs.

GLUE SNIFFING and inhalation of organic solvents such as butane, and those in some hair sprays and lighter fuels, is practised mainly by the 14 and 15 year-old age group. In one survey, seven per cent admitted that they had tried these drugs at some time, and of these 19 per cent were smokers. An American survey found cases of lung damage and irregular heart beats among 'sniffers'. Sniffing is attractive to some people because of its effects on the central nervous system, and the feelings it brings of exhilaration, euphoria, some hallucinations and a sense of 'insight'. Side effects include depression in some cases, anxiety states, and distortion of thinking. Liver damage has been reported in a few instances and there have been several fatalities.

HALLUCINOGENS such as LSD and DOM produce effects similar to solvent inhaling, but more marked. (LSD stands for a synthetic organic compound named Lysergic acid.) They are swallowed and produce feelings of 'insight', distortion of sensations leading to hallucinations, and a mood of exhilaration. Side effects physically include rapid heart rate, raised blood pressure and muscle weakness; mentally, the regular user may develop severe psychiatric symptoms (psychosis), as well as anxiety, depression, and sometimes homicidal or suicidal feelings.

OPIOIDS include morphine injections, papaveratum taken orally or by injection, nepenthe, laudanum (opium tincture), and heroin (diamorphine) taken by injection or as tablets. The desired effects are tranquillity, euphoria, 'Nirvana', together with sleep and very pleasant dreams (Morpheus was the God of Dreams). Side effects which Cystic Fibrosis people should note are loss of appetite, respiratory depression and suppression of coughing.

COCAINE and its synthetic derivative are used for central nervous system stimulation. The rebound side effects can be serious.

Any of these drugs will, in time, have potentially serious physical toxic effects, in addition to the well-known psychiatric and personality problems. The physical effects of toxicity, which Cystic Fibrosis people especially should consider are:

1   *Reduced appetite* with lowered food consumption and consequent protein and vitamin deficiencies, leading to relative malnutrition and an impaired ability to cope with chest infections; there will also be muscle weakness and general debility. This applies to solvent sniffing, opioids, cocaine, benzodiazapines, amphetamines and alcohol excess. Cannabis usually lowers the appetite, but is said sometimes to induce temporary spells of heavy eating.

2   Very important *effects on bronchial tubes* and *lungs* are reported with opioids, cannabis, some benzodiazapines, and alcohol abuse.

3   *Cirrhosis of the liver* (Multilobular type) is widely recognised as a common, very serious complication of continued alcohol abuse. Some degree of liver damage is also reported in addiction to solvents and some sedative drugs, including benzodiazapines. Alcohol abuse may also cause *pancreatitis* and so probably damage any residual pancreatic function in Cystic Fibrosis.

    Hepatitis B may be caught by users of hypodermic needles, which are often shared by several people or even a group of opioid addicts.

4   *A general lowering of resistance* to infections is frequently
encountered in all forms of continued drug taking.
Hypodermic needles shared among drugs users can
transmit something even more serious than Hepatitis B,
something which threatens to become epidemic in various parts of the world and is referred to in general terms
as AIDS. This requires a section to itself.

Aids

This is a word like NATO (North Atlantic Treaty Organisation), whose letters are the initials of the words describing
what it stands for.

A = *Acquired*, to distinguish it from inborn, inherited
I = *Immune*, affecting the body's defence system
D = *Deficiency* (of a vital part of this immune mechanism)
S = *Syndrome*: a group of symptoms of disease states going
      together, characteristic of a particular problem

AIDS is the end stage, after a variable period of time,
of infection with a particular virus (HIV, or Human
Immunodeficiency Virus), which disables certain specialised cells forming a very important part of the body's
defence system. The symptoms include progressive general debility and loss of weight, pneumonia due to unusual
bacteria, viruses and parasitic organisms, together with
enlarged liver, spleen and glands. The brain may be
affected, and various forms of cancer are often the terminal
disease.

It is not yet known for certain how many people in the
United States and Europe have been infected by the HIV,
nor what proportion of these have gone on to develop
AIDS—estimates from various centres range fron ten to 40
per cent. The latent period is also not fully understood;
studies of homosexual men gave a time interval ranging
from two to seven years from HIV to AIDS, but with
increasing experience both these estimates will probably
need revision.

What is known is that the incidence of AIDS is increasing and that it remains, at present, incurable.

Cystic Fibrosis people can therefore appreciate how vitally important it is NOT to get infected with the HIV and so NOT to get AIDS. Although at present AIDS is thought to be relatively rare among sexually active teenagers, it is just as well for Cystic Fibrosis people to be prepared.

The commonest way in which the AIDS is transmitted is by promiscuous sexual behaviour. When the problem first came to the fore, it appeared among homosexuals, especially communities where promiscuity was common; now, however, although it seems that male homosexuals are still at the greatest risk, AIDS is appearing more frequently among heterosexuals.

Another route for the spread of AIDS is via the sharing of needles by drug addicts. Some blood products needed by haemophilia patients (for example, Factor VIII) were found to contain the virus and a number of haemophiliacs became infected. This has been rectified, and the blood factors needed by these patients are now quite safe. The virus has also been isolated from human milk, from saliva, and tears. There have been a few reports in the American press of AIDS cases allegedly resulting from 'wet kissing', but to date I have found no evidence to confirm this.

Free condoms have been issued to first year students at one provincial university in the United Kingdom, in the hope of preventing both AIDS and unwanted pregnancies. The condom, properly used, is a reasonably effective contraceptive, and certainly minimises the risk of contracting AIDS, but is not completely foolproof.

The only certain way to avoid AIDS is to have and to hold one sexual partner for life.

Fertility

When considering physical growth and sexual maturity in Cystic Fibrosis teenagers, we learned that in a number of girls puberty was delayed by about two years, but that eventually menstruation and the physical signs of puberty developed normally. We saw also that the thick, viscid mucus in the uterine cervix could impede the entrance and penetration by sperm. Another factor sometimes reducing fertility (perhaps only temporary) could be irregular production of eggs by the ovaries, usually associated with poor nutrition and below-average weight.

Cystic Fibrosis females are by no means infertile—about 100 have conceived and given birth. Pregnancy, however, should not be considered lightly: a careful and exhaustive review of the woman's health is essential. After all, pregnancy exerts some strain on most organs and should only be contemplated by a Cystic Fibrosis woman with a high clinical score on the Shwachman scale or similar, good nutritional condition and weight, good lung function (at least 60 per cent), and without any significant complications.

What about the adolescent Cystic Fibrosis girl? The unplanned, unwanted pregnancy could obviously be a disaster of the first magnitude. I should therefore like to offer some advice on contraception, which applies equally to the adult Cystic Fibrosis woman. What should you look for in a contraceptive method? Effectiveness, acceptability and freedom from significant side effects are the three essentials. I shall consider the Pill, intra-uterine devices, and other barrier techniques. (These are covered in health education in the fourth and fifth years at some comprehensive schools, where the curriculum also includes alcohol, drug abuse and AIDS.)

The *Combined Oral Contraceptive* (The Pill) is the most effective preparation. It contains two female hormones (oestrogen 30–50 micrograms, and progesterone). They act by inhibiting ovulation and the 30 microgram one is usually suitable for Cystic Fibrosis women. Some fears have been raised regarding the effects of medicines which the patient may be taking, including antibiotics such as Ampicillin. The general medical consensus is that antibiotics do not interfere with absorption unless they cause vomiting or diarrhoea.

There is a small risk of blood clots forming in the veins where high oestrogen content pills (50 micrograms) are combined with cigarette smoking. The usual mild diabetes and minimal liver involvement are not considered bars against taking what is, after all, the most effective contraceptive apart from sterilisation. Most Cystic Fibrosis females are in fact advised to avoid pregnancy altogether.

Alternatives are *intra-uterine devices* such as the coil, generally considered unsuitable for women who have not borne a child, and *barrier methods*, such as a cap, diaphragm or condom. I would suggest that if for any reason the oral contraceptive is not suitable, then a condom together with a spermicidal preparation (cream, gel, or foam), or pessaries such as Rendells, would make the next best combined technique.

I make no apology for reiterating that pregnancy in Cystic Fibrosis women requires careful thought, consultations with the Cystic Fibrosis specialist and possibly other colleagues, followed by planned monitoring of the pregnancy and delivery of the baby in hospital after pre-natal admission for preparatory care and therapy.

Some of the adolescents I have mentioned in this and the previous chapter are now in different medical care ('a grown-up doctor', as one mother told me). In many places the transfer from the paediatric clinic to an adult Cystic Fibrosis clinic takes place when the teenager reaches the age of 16.

As I have emphasised in the text so far, the maintenance of optimal lung function during childhood is essential for adolescence to be a time of growth and development in all their aspects—physical, sexual and psychosocial. During adolescence the change from being dependent and having to be cared for, to achieving independence in daily living and learning how to become truly adult, also means maintaining the best possible health of the respiratory tract.

In a paper produced in 1986, Dr Margaret Mearns followed a group of adolescents (13–20 year-olds) at Queen Elizabeth Hospital for Children and found that 63 per cent had achieved good lung function, with no cough and the potential for normal activity. A further 21 per cent had near-normal activity, with a 'productive cough'. These results are encouraging.

Ideally, the transfer from paediatric to adult medical care should be effected by an extension of the 'shared care' system which I have described previously. Initially, a doctor with an interest in Cystic Fibrosis—probably a chest physician—would attend the regular check-up sessions held at a regional Cystic Fibrosis centre, get to know the adolescents and follow their progress. Following the official transfer to an adult Cystic Fibrosis unit, when they would join the Association of Cystic Fibrosis Adults, one of the paediatricians familiar with the patients would attend the new clinic from time to time.

9 CYSTIC FIBROSIS IN ADULTHOOD

Several recent surveys put the number of known sufferers from Cystic Fibrosis in the United Kingdom at around 6,000. In a debate in the House of Commons in December 1987, Mr Ivan Lawrence, MP for Burton, speaking in favour of prescription charge exemption for Cystic Fibrosis sufferers, said that there were at that time some 5,600 Cystic Fibrosis sufferers in the United Kingdom, increasing annually by between 200 and 300. He quoted a figure of 2,400 Cystic Fibrosis sufferers over the age of 16—those not included for exemption from prescription charges.

I shall return to this welfare subject later. In the meantime, there are some further estimates of the numbers of Cystic Fibrosis adolescents and adults for us to consider. The Association of Cystic Fibrosis Adults (UK) estimated in 1987 that there were 1,300 people with Cystic Fibrosis over the age of 16, with a further 100 adults accruing annually, and that by 1990 there would be an extra 1,000 adolescent Cystic Fibrosis boys and girls.

Reports from the Medical Research Council and the British Paediatric Association give similar figures, and recently Professor John Dodge forecast that by the year 2000 there will be 6,500 Cystic Fibrosis sufferers in the United Kingdom Computer Database, with over 1,000 aged between ten and fourteen and 200 per year entering the adult Cystic Fibrosis group.

These findings, together with the growing impact of the Association of Cystic Fibrosis Adults (UK) and associated international Cystic Fibrosis groups, reflect the remarkable improvement over the past 25 years, due to research, in life expectancy and quality; as was said in Parliament, this owes much to the ongoing support of the Cystic Fibrosis Research Trust.

Facts and Figures

My information is drawn from various sources: the Association of Cystic Fibrosis Adults (UK) and the Cystic Fibrosis Foundation (USA) with clinical data from two large adult Cystic Fibrosis centres, one in the United Kingdom, the other in the United States.

STATISTICAL INFORMATION ON ADULTS WITH
CYSTIC FIBROSIS

1987	UNITED KINGDOM	UNITED STATES
Estimated total CF patients	6,000	30,000
Number of adults (over 16 years)	1,300	7,000
Age range	16–49	16–41
Mean Age	22	22
Percentage in employment	50%	80%
	Clerical, technical and management = 45%	All fields of employment
	Skilled artisans = 30%	
	Professions = 25%	
Students (sixth form, college, university)	16–30%	Research students rated as employed
Housewives	5–16%	Many in part-time jobs; some working from home
Unemployed	20%	

Health matters		
General rating (based on internationally agreed score)	Mild 35%	Mild 35%
	Moderate 50%	Moderate 45%
	Severe 15%	Severe 20%

Meconium ileus equivalent	20% (less frequent and severe since 1983)	10% Group presenting with MI at birth, follow-up showed no long-term effect

1987	UNITED KINGDOM	UNITED STATES
Diabetes	12%	10%
	(4% need Insulin)	(8% on Insulin)
	(No serious complications)	(No serious complications)
Liver and biliary problems:		
(cirrhosis)	5%	5%
severe symptoms	less than 2%	less than 2%

There is little doubt that the steadily increasing cohort of adult Cystic Fibrosis patients necessitates the establishment of Special Care centres similar to, possibly combined with, the regional Cystic Fibrosis centre. Such a unit has been in operation for more than twenty years at the Brompton Hospital, London, with Sir John Batten and his team of specialists in general and thoracic medicine and allied disciplines.

The results from this exemplary institution, together with those from similar units being established in the United Kingdom and in Australia, the United States and Canada, show beyond doubt that not only the length of life but the degree of health and happiness for these patients is greatly enhanced.

Although I have had very little personal experience of the care of adult Cystic Fibrosis patients, I have seen enough of the work being done in these Special Care centres to feel that I can offer an opinion on the needs of this group of patients.

Your motto could be 'self care—shared care'. What do you have a right to expect, and what should you do in order to get the best results?

You are entitled to up-to-date and continuing expert medical service from doctors and other medical colleagues as necessary, who will be in touch with all recent developments in Cystic Fibrosis. You should have regular medical assessments and should be able to contact members of the medical care team if any problem arises which gives you cause for concern. Your treatment should be non-regimented, but individualised, according to your needs and circumstances and your ability to cope with Cystic Fibrosis. You may require admission to hospital for treatment of your lung infection or some complication. If so, you need a relaxed hospital environment, with a single or shared room if possible, avoidance of tobacco smoke, and available medical and paramedical staff. As a corollary of this, as much of your treatment as possible should be done at home.

You know by now that care of the respiratory tract is all-important. This includes physiotherapy, antibiotics taken intravenously, orally or by nebuliser, and regular physical exercise. Complementary care includes attention to nutrition, with a high calorie, high protein diet, and correct doses of the most suitable pancreatic extracts.

These things you can see to yourself. I know that physiotherapy can seem a boring chore, especially when it has to be done for twenty minutes at least twice a day—in the early morning and then again before the evening meal —but you must train yourself to do the forced expiration technique, postural drainage and breathing exercises. These techniques will have been taught you by the Cystic Fibrosis centre, and you should verify at your regular check-up visits that you are doing the job correctly. If you could only see, as I have done, the improvement in pulmonary function tests produced by the combination of regular, effective physiotherapy with regular daily exercise or games, then you would train yourself and dedicate time and effort to it. The good results will be reflected in less frequent and less severe pseudomonas flare-ups and so less frequent hospital admission for intensive treatment.

Digestive and Abdominal Symptoms
From information which I have gathered from a number of different sources, I would say that at least one quarter of Cystic Fibrosis adults have abdominal symptoms at some time or another. This section is intended to be an outline of the main causes of alimentary tract troubles, particularly the various kinds of pain or discomfort, the different regions where pain is felt, and what you should do about it.

Some of the information given below has already been discussed in Chapter Eight, but I raise it again here, in an adult context, because of its importance.

Probably the commonest type of abdominal pain is that termed by doctors 'colicky abdominal pain'. This means pain coming on in waves, rising to a peak of intensity, then subsiding, and so recurring in cycles for a variable period of time. The pain is felt as cramp-like; sometimes the peak intensity makes you feel sick or even vomit and feel faint. If you put your hand on the painful area it is not usually very tender, and warmth, from a hot water bottle, for instance, may give temporary relief.

Colicky pain is caused by spasms in the muscular wall of some hollow or tube-like structure somewhere in the abdomen. You should note and tell the doctor exactly where you felt the pain at the onset, and whether it radiated to any other part. Figure 6 illustrates some of the commoner sites where colicky pains occur, and this gives some indication of what organ is likely to be affected.

A common site where colicky abdominal pain may begin is A in the diagram, in the centre of the abdomen, around the navel. This indicates some disturbance in the small intestine—either an inflammation connected with this part of the gut, or some block in the passage of the bowel contents through the small gut (where they are normally fluid) into the large intestine where the bowel contents become semi-solid and 'formed'. As the pain continues, it may also be felt at G in the lower left quarter of the abdomen, caused by spasmodic attempts of the large bowel to evacuate its contents. In other cases, the central colicky pains persist and are accompanied by nausea and distension of the central part of the abdomen; later by vomiting, which may be continual. These are all typical symptoms of meconium ileus equivalent, which, as I pointed out in Chapter Eight, has nothing to do with meconium but is due to intestinal obstruction by faecal matter with un-digested fat, sticky mucus and generally thick, tenacious undigested matter which is too difficult for the muscular waves (peristalsis) to move along.

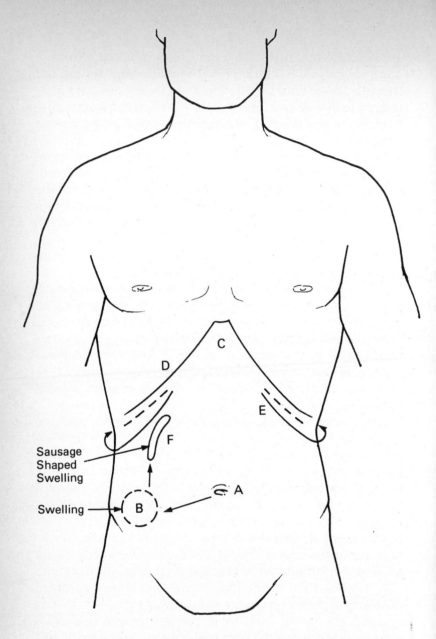

Figure 6. Causes of abdominal pain in Cystic Fibrosis adults. A = intestinal colic (meconium ileus equivalent). B = further stage of A, and also appendicitis. C and D = gall bladder infection, gall stones. E = pancreatitis. F = intussusception.

This condition occurs in a mild form in about a third of adult Cystic Fibrosis sufferers. The pain is not severe and the attacks are short-lived: sometimes they are obviously related to one or two large meals without a corresponding increase in the dose of Pancreatin, a situation easily put right.

In some instances, however, the symptoms are more severe, as described above. The pain shifts from the centre of the abdomen (point A) to the right lower part of the abdomen (point B in the diagram), and you may feel a swelling in that area, usually only slightly tender, if at all. This is a situation which needs urgent medical investigation and treatment, and you should report right away with an account of the symptoms as mentioned above.

Meconium ileus equivalent is really a type of intestinal obstruction due to the abnormal contents of the bowel, and affects especially the lower part of the small intestine and the colon, hence the alternative title DIOS—distal intestinal obstruction syndrome. You will hear or read these medical terms, so you should know what it is all about, so that you can give the doctors an accurate account of your symptoms.

One reason for urgent assessment must have come to mind already—the possibility of appendicitis with an abscess, which can occur in anybody (Cystic Fibrosis or not) in the teenage and young adult group. You would, however, notice marked tenderness around point B. A second reason is that, if neglected, DIOS may eventually require surgery. This is to be avoided if at all possible.

Treatment at the present time comprises hospital admission for intravenous fluids, pain relieving medicine, a naso-gastric tube for suction and special solutions to liquefy the plasticine-like contents of the intestine—Airbron, Diatbizoate, or Gastrografin by intestinal tube and enemas under X-ray control. Following an acute attack, mucus-liquefying medicine is taken orally for several weeks, and a review of your diet and Pancreatin therapy will be organised. Proper doses of modern enteric-coated microspheres (Creon or Pancrease) should avoid relapses.

Another, much less common but nevertheless important condition, is intussusception. This is a condition which paediatricians are accustomed to diagnose and treat in small children, especially boys, between three months and two years of age. The common variety is called ileo-colic, in which the end portion of the small intestine (the ileum) become telescoped into the beginning of the large gut (the caecum). This happens near the appendix (see Figure 4, p. 115), which is why it can be difficult at first to distinguish between intussusception and appendicitis. The process of intussusception can go on and on through the large gut and occasionally it can come out through the anus, rather like the rectal prolapse described earlier, which is common in Cystic Fibrosis children and a factor in the diagnosis.

In older teenage and young adult patients, intussusception may be a complication of the MIE/DIOS condition, although the pain is usually quite severe and a lump can be felt in some area of the large gut, a tender sausage-shaped swelling. In younger patients blood may be passed through the anus. If the condition is diagnosed early enough (X-ray with barium enema is required) it can sometimes be reduced by the barium without the need for surgery.

Other causes of abdominal symptoms in young adults are:

1   *Gallstones*, which were found in ten per cent of one series of patients in the United States but do not often cause symptoms. Pain is felt at point D in Figure 6, and may radiate round to the back.
2   Inflammation of the pancreas (pancreatitis) occasionally occurs in older patients, with pain in the C-E region, again radiating round the left flank to the back.
3   Duodenal ulcer.

Care of the Respiratory System
Recently, there have been trials of newer drugs and respiratory techniques in the hope of improving the treatment of the common pseudomonas bacterial infection in the lungs, and perhaps other parts of the respiratory tract. I shall

consider these under the two main headings of lung care —antibiotics and physiotherapy.

Antibiotics

Oral antibiotics used to be available for treatment of Cystic Fibrosis lung infection in babies and children, when the trouble was caused by the staphylococcus germ. Flucloxacillin, a type of penicillin effective even against resistant staphylococcal germs, can be given orally as capsules or syrup (Floxapen) for prevention and treatment, over short or long periods as the doctors consider necessary. This was very effective. Unfortunately, over the past decade the newer type of infection with the pseudomonas germ has come in, even in infancy, and is certainly the most common infection in adults. This germ is very difficult to eradicate but it can be kept under control by intensive treatment, which usually means admission to hospital for several weeks, three or four times a year.

For the patients, however, going into hospital for several weeks can be difficult and disruptive. Students working for 'A' levels or college and university examinations find it very awkward, as it is for those in some jobs. Therefore we would all like as much treatment as possible to be carried out at home (some of it would very likely be required at your place of work or study). The standard treatment for pseudomonas infection is intravenous injections (drip, or bolus—one shot at a time) which can be given at home in appropriate cases. Your advisers in the clinic will assess your suitability and, if you are all agreed, will fit you with an indwelling vein cannula (tube). It is important that provision should be made for immediate help should the cannula become blocked. Sometimes your own doctor can clear it, or the casualty department at the local hospital. Failing these, you must be able to go at once to the regional unit. You must keep the telephone numbers of all these handy.

The intravenous antibiotics normally used are combinations, such as a penicillin (for example, azlocillin) with one of the aminoglycosides (for example, gentamycin). Recent trials with a newer, different type of antibiotic known as ceftazidime indicate that this drug is very useful against pseudomonas infection which is not responding well to the customary treatment. Some Cystic Fibrosis centres are using it as a first-line antibiotic. You will be advised and instructed on all these matters.

Two recent investigations should be mentioned here. First, the new antibiotic ciprofloxacin, which is not only very effective against the usual strains of pseudomonas (including the mucoid type) but can be given orally, which is obviously a great advantage for those in work or studying. The best treatment schedule for ciprofloxacin is not yet quite agreed, but most centres advise short courses between administrations of the standard antibiotics.

The second development is in nebulisation aerosol treatment, using the favoured combination of antibiotics such as gentamycin and azlocillin. It is important that you have the correct type of nebuliser, capable of delivering the required volume of aerosol with the desired proportion of very small droplets, so that the antibiotics may penetrate the small bronchial tubes deep in the lung tissue. Recent controlled trials of nebulisation treatment have shown that, properly done, it can provide a valuable contribution to respiratory tract care. The aerosol with antibiotics is to be used after physiotherapy has cleared the sputum from the airways; sometimes an aerosol is used before physiotherapy, but then it carries something to help liquefy the sticky mucus or to relax a bronchial spasm which is producing wheezing.

Thus, both oral ciproflaxin and aerosol nebulised antibiotics should help greatly in controlling the difficult pseudomonas.

Physiotherapy
The prime importance, in fact essential need, for effective physiotherapy is emphasised yet again. This, more than anything else, is in my opinion your self care in operation. The Cystic Fibrosis Research Trust publishes an excellent booklet, *The Physical Treatment of Cystic Fibrosis*, written by leading experts in the field, which I strongly urge you to

read and follow. It shows you how, by self-discipline, it is possible to achieve most of the aims of physiotherapy on your own, so allowing you a greater degree of independence. It is essential, however, to keep in touch with your physiotherapist at the Cystic Fibrosis centre.

Something called the PEP mask has been in the Cystic Fibrosis papers recently. This stands for 'positive expiratory pressure' and the idea behind it is that if you have some trouble with your bronchial tubes, when you breathe out the small airways will tend to collapse, so that you will not be able to cough up the mucus from that part of your lungs. If you breathe out against a pressure, this will tend to keep the small bronchial tubes open, so that coughing just afterwards will get rid of the pent-up sputum (containing infected sputum) from the distant parts of the lung.

Several trials of PEP have been reported at recent international conferences. A few investigators found that the PEP mask (used at home) appeared to be beneficial, but a controlled scientific trial of the Brompton Hospital group showed that breathing exercises (emphasising inspiration), interspersed with the forced expiratory technique and postural drainage (that is BE + FET + PD in the Cystic Fibrosis jargon you are accustomed to hear), gave just as good results as PEP.

When I listened to a discussion on this in Israel a few years ago, I was reminded of a time, many years back, when I worked in a hospital to which was attached a special ward for miners suffering from that dread occupational disease silicosis. There was a pleasant balcony attached to the ward, with views over the sea to Devon, and the patients would sit and gaze and wheeze, chat and cough for many hours, with oxygen cylinders, masks and sputum cups to hand. I often went to chat to them about non-medical matters, and was intrigued to see most of them breathing in a laboured way, but pursing their lips when breathing out—a sort of silent whistling. They told me this was something they had picked up in the coal mines from fellow workers who had 'a touch of the dust' and found this silent whistling technique, followed by coughing, helped to clear the tubes. One old chap with blue lips showed me how he did it, coughed up some yellow phlegm, then put on the oxygen mask and inhaled for a minute or so. He was obviously relieved and his lips were a better colour. This was evidently a kind of PEP combined with FET, I should think. The ward grew and subsequently became the world-famous Pneumoconiosis Research Unit of the Medical Research Council.

Allowances, Benefits and Welfare
In the last chapter I dealt briefly with some aspects of employment and training, mainly for school leavers, through the officers of the Careers Guidance Service. At present the choice is between finding a job, entering the Youth Training Scheme, further education, and un-employment.

I also described the help available from the Job Centre and the associated Disablement Resettlement Officer, together with some of the financial allowances which you can claim. Altogether these comprise Sickness Benefit, Invalidity Benefit (contributory, or indirectly so), and Severe Disablement Allowance. You may also claim Mobil-ity Allowance or Invalid Care Allowance, Income Support and special additional loans and grants from the Social Fund. All these are described in the booklet, *Guide to Government and Voluntary Help*, obtainable from the Cystic Fibrosis Research Trust.

Social Security Welfare Benefits
Income Support is intended to meet regular weekly needs, and parents and patients should be able to get help for the extra expenses involved in caring for someone with Cystic Fibrosis. It may be claimed by those who are unemployed, bringing up children on their own, too disabled to work or only able to work part time, or staying at home to look after a disabled relative. Those in work for 24 hours or more per week are not normally eligible unless they are so disabled that their earnings are too little to live on.

Those on Income Support do not have to pay for any of the following, whether for themselves, their partners or their children: NHS prescriptions, NHS dental treatment, travel to hospital for NHS treatment. They may also get help with the cost of spectacles. Those Cystic Fibrosis people who for one reason or another cannot claim for the NHS prescription charge should consider using a 'season ticket', which involves paying in advance for four or twelve months at a discount. However, increasing pressure on the Government by members of all parties raises hopes that Cystic Fibrosis will be included in the list of exempted chronic illnesses, such as Diabetes.

You may also be able to get some help from the Social Fund—for a new baby, funeral expenses or other exceptional calls on your funds. These single payment or urgent payment needs are made from a fixed annual budget in the form of grants or loans. Claimants have no legal entitlement to either a grant or a loan, but funds may be available in exceptional cases—for example, for extra heating, special expensive dietary needs (extra rich high calories supplements, in line with the new thinking about Cystic Fibrosis food requirements), and laundry and clothing wear and tear, in view of frequent soiling. Certain necessary adaptations to rooms for physiotherapy, nebuliser therapy and ventilation may be funded, and Housing Benefit from the Local Council is available.

Children, adolescents and adults with Cystic Fibrosis are covered under the scheme. In addition to allowances for single persons, couples and parents , extra premiums cater for families, child disability (Attendance Allowance equivalent), single parents, invalidity and mobility allowances. Special allowances for disabled students are also available.

Further information and advice may be sought from your local Citizens' Advice Bureau, or from your Social Security office where you can also obtain leaflets relating to these benefits: SB20 *A Guide to Income Support*, FB23 *Young People's Guide*, FB27 *Bringing Up Children*, and FB28 *Sick or Disabled*.

The Welfare Officer of the Cystic Fibrosis Research Trust will assist you in many ways. If you wish to write to her, the address is: Cystic Fibrosis Research Trust, Welfare Department, Alexandra House, 5 Blyth Road, Bromley, Kent BR1 3RS. Please give as many details of your case and circumstances as possible: full names and dates of birth of Cystic Fibrosis patients, time spent on physiotherapy, what medicines, such as antibiotics and aerosols, you have to give or supervise, and all the attention and extra chores you have by day and at night. You should also state how far you have to travel to attend your regional Cystic Fibrosis clinic (give name and address) and how often you have to go there.

The recent introduction of the Cystic Fibrosis Nurse Clinical Specialist to the group at some Cystic Fibrosis regional centres has already proved a most welcome and effective project. By this appointment, an experienced professional liaison officer fits into the team with the social workers, doctors, physiotherapists, dieticians and home and community health care personnel. This professional help will be available to you at home, with friendly, helpful and expert advice on many problems, including welfare.

Travelling Abroad
On several occasions I have been asked about the advisability of travel abroad for Cystic Fibrosis people. Air travel should be no problem, except for those few with severe lung trouble, who require oxygen: such patients should discuss the matter with their Cystic Fibrosis unit and the airline concerned.

Holidays abroad are in order, but you should carry a letter setting out your treatment needs and current state of health; you should also know the address of the Cystic Fibrosis organisation in your country of holiday travel. A list of the European centres is given below. The DSS local office has two helpful leaflets, SA30 and SA35, dealing with journeys abroad.

*European and Neighbouring Countries, Associated with the
International Cystic Fibrosis Association and the European
Working Group for Cystic Fibrosis*

Austrian Cystic Fibrosis Association, University Kinder-
klimk, Vienna.

Belgian Association for Cystic Fibrosis, Brussels.

Czech Pediatric Society Cystic Fibrosis Committee, Prague.

Danish Cystic Fibrosis Association, Viborg.

Eire: Cystic Fibrosis Association of Ireland, Dublin.

West Germany: Cystic Fibrosis Association, Nürnberg.

East Germany: Cystic Fibrosis Working Group, Dresden.

Finland: Cystic Fibrosis Association, Helsinki.

France: Cystic Fibrosis Association, Paris.

Greece: Hellenic Cystic Fibrosis Association, Athens.

Hungary: National Working Group Cystic Fibrosis,
University Szeged.

Iceland: Cystic Fibrosis Group, Reykjavik.

Israel: Cystic Fibrosis Foundation of Israel, Tel Aviv.

Italy: Cystic Fibrosis Association, Venice.

Netherlands: National Cystic Fibrosis Association, Utrecht.

Norway: Cystic Fibrosis Association, Oslo.

Poland: National Research Institute, Warsaw.

Portugal: Cystic Fibrosis Group, Oeiras.

Spain: Cystic Fibrosis Association, Barcelona.

Sweden: Association for Cystic Fibrosis, Uppsala.

Switzerland: Cystic Fibrosis Association, Utendorf.

United Kingdom: (GB) Cystic Fibrosis Research Trust,
Bromley.

Yugoslavia: Cystic Fibrosis in Mother and Child Institute,
Belgrade.

Also, now associated with the European Group and
sharing experience of Cystic Fibrosis:

USSR: Academy of Medical Sciences, Moscow.

Accumulated statistics from this multinational group
suggest the following approximate figures:

a) Carriers of the Cystic Fibrosis gene in Europe = 14–15
million.

b) Number of Cystic Fibrosis babies born annually = 1,700.

10 TRANSPLANT SURGERY FOR CYSTIC FIBROSIS

To those of us who are amateur gardeners, the word 'transplant' evokes memories of lifting small plants from seed pots or boxes and planting them out in chosen places in our gardens. More experienced friends may tell us that the notion of transplanting includes grafting a portion of one plant or even animal onto another plant or animal, so that the two unite organically.

Human skin grafting techniques became progressively developed during the Second World War, saving the lives and sanity of many badly injured people in the Armed Forces and among the civilian population. Human kidney transplantation has been successfully carried out in the United Kingdom since the 1960s.

Transplantation of the human heart, at first only partially successful, became an established method of treatment during the 1970s, followed by liver transplants. Then, in the 1980s, heart-and-lung transplantation was developed for certain diseases affecting these organs. By the end of 1987, 150 operations for transplanting heart and lungs had been carried out by the specialist units at Papworth and Harefield Hospitals and, since 1985, 16 of those heart/lung transplants had been performed for patients with Cystic Fibrosis.

It has been known for a long time that some patients suffering from chronic lung trouble such as bronchitis, emphysema, silicosis and similar disorders may eventually develop a form of heart disease. This also applies to Cystic Fibrosis. In a few cases, despite regular intensive treatment with antibiotics, physiotherapy, breathing and general exercises, nebulisers and proper nutritional care, the lung trouble persists inexorably. In time the extra strain all this imposes upon the heart begins to tell, and it is for patients like this that transplantation of heart and lungs may be life-saving.

Transplantation of the heart and the lungs is a new development in this remarkable field of major surgery, due largely to the skill and dedication of Professor Yacoub and Mr John Wallwork. The overall techniques involved still carry significant risks, partly from the operation itself and partly from the problems of rejection, when the body's immune defence system detects the entry of foreign protein material and triggers off its natural responses aimed at eliminating the invader. This rejection phenomenon has been treated by various 'immuno-suppressive' drugs such as azothioprine, and by corticosteroids such as predniso-lone. The drugs not only suppress rejection of the trans-planted organs but interfere with the body's resistance to infections, causing bone marrow toxic effects; great care is therefore required in protecting the patient while the treatment is continuing.

In the case of patients with Cystic Fibrosis, who are in any case liable to lung infection, the surgeons were at first understandably cautious about undertaking such a major procedure. There was also concern that the unknown in-trinsic basic defect in Cystic Fibrosis, which leads to defec-tive mucus-ciliary lung clearance, might still be operative in the transplanted lungs, and that the disease would develop again in these organs.

The introduction of a new drug, cyclosporin (Sandim-mun) which is a powerful antidote to organ transplant rejection and virtually free from toxic effects on the bone marrow, brought increased confidence. In October 1985 the first heart/lungs transplant for Cystic Fibrosis was carried out.

Cystic Fibrosis patients who are considered by their doctors to be possibly suitable for heart and lungs trans-plant, and would like to go ahead with the project, are first subjected to a detailed hospital assessment taking several weeks. Following this, if the findings are satisfactory, they are referred to one of the transplant surgeons at his hospital in Cambridge, Harefield, Middlesex, or Brompton Hospital in London. While waiting for a suitable donor, the patient must do everything he or she can to remain as fit and well as possible, in consultation with the local Cystic Fibrosis centre. Then, immediately a suitable transplant is known to be available, the patient must be taken without delay to the transplant hospital. The post-operative hospital stay is likely to be a month or so, followed by daily treatment at home and visits to the out-patient clinic at regular intervals, frequent at first, then gradually changing to three-monthly. All reasonable steps to avoid infection must be taken, and any symptoms such as headache, sore throat, cough, pain in the chest, a rash or painful joint, should be reported straight away. These intermittent infections will respond to treatment with antibiotics if taken early.

Occasional instances of rejection can occur. Such symptoms as feeling generally unwell, loss of appetite, weakness and lethargy, or loss of weight, may herald an emergency, and the patient must be readmitted to hospital for further treatment with, perhaps, cyclosporin and corticosteroids. The rejection crisis will soon be under control.

'This is all very well,' one patient said to me, 'but I'd still have Cystic Fibrosis, wouldn't I? My new lungs could get infected by the pseudomonas again, or legionnaire's disease, as I heard about the other day. My digestion wouldn't work any better, I'd still have to take my Pancreatin capsules and the gastric tablets' (he meant Cimetidine or Ranitidine), 'and I could still get Diabetes.'

There is of course something in what he said. The clinical and biochemical markers of Cystic Fibrosis will remain —the sweat still abnormally salty, the 'Cystic Fibrosis factor' in the blood still positive, and the likelihood of sinusitis and polyps if he had them previously. His digestion and nutrition should, however, improve. There is a reciprocal relationship between the lungs and digestive function: if lung problems increase, pancreatic efficiency deteriorates. When close attention is given to diet, and pancreatic supplements, the lung problems decrease and health generally is better.

In any case, there is as yet no sign of pulmonary infections of the Cystic Fibrosis type in the patients who have had heart/lung transplants and have been monitored for up to two-and-a-half years. Obviously there is a need for continuous and long-term follow-up before we can be sure.

What we must bear in mind is the overall strategy. The aim is to find a 'cure' for Cystic Fibrosis, or a new drug treatment which will control the disease in the way that Insulin controls Diabetes, thyroxine replaces and controls the inborn error of cretinism, and special diet controls the metabolic congenital abnormality in Phenylketonuria (PKU) for which we screen newborn babies—just as some of us would like to screen all new babies for Cystic Fibrosis. So, while we await the solution of this problem, heart/lung transplantation may afford a new lease of life.

Most of the information in this chapter has been drawn from the article by Dr Margaret Hodson in the Winter 1987 issue of the *Cystic Fibrosis News*, published by the Cystic Fibrosis Research Trust. I should like to express my thanks for permission to use this review, and finish with a summary of the admirable and heart-warming case featured in the paper.

Miss Julie Bennett had the heart/lungs transplant operation in October 1985. Her life-style and social activities had been severely limited by Cystic Fibrosis. Now, two years after the operation, she is working full time and walks two to three miles daily. Like others who have had successful heart/lung transplants, she may, one hopes, look forward to greater activity—walking, running, dancing and holidays abroad. The Cystic Fibrosis heart/lung transplant endeavour is supported by the Cystic Fibrosis Research Trust to the extent of half a million pounds.

11   *LOOKING INTO THE FUTURE*

Cystic Fibrosis was put on the map medically, so to speak, just half a century ago, although I have no doubt the condition has been with us for very much longer—possibly ten or twelve thousand years. In that half-century it has attracted increasing attention, with cheering results. Figure 7 shows how the outlook for Cystic Fibrosis patients has improved, particularly over the past decade with the setting up of Cystic Fibrosis centres. Today, about three-quarters of patients can expect to reach adulthood. Not only that, but they can look forward to independent life-styles, careers, jobs, friends and marriage. The medical treatment now available, with powerful antibiotics aided by up-to-date physiotherapy and backed by the new thinking regarding nutrition and diet, are largely responsible for this greatly improved outlook.

Much, however, remains to be done, for there is still no cure for Cystic Fibrosis. Active research is pursuing several lines of enquiry, and it seems appropriate to conclude by looking at some of these.

Research into Cystic Fibrosis
Until about ten years ago, most research projects were orientated towards the 'mucoviscidosis' notion of Cystic Fibrosis. There is no doubt that the mucus secretions in the lungs are unusually thick and sticky, and that the pancreatic ducts appear to be blocked by very thick secretions. Investigations studied the chemical composition of mucus, including complex carbohydrates, but got no further towards identifying the long-sought 'basic defect'.

While studying the bronchial mucus glands and their secretion, however, some researchers noticed that the

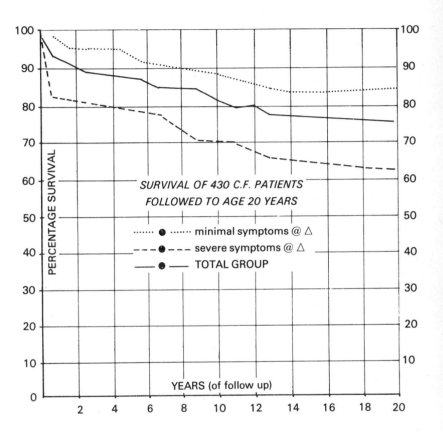

Figure 7. Survival of 430 Cystic Fibrosis patients followed to the age of 20.

ciliary clearance mechanism appeared defective in Cystic Fibrosis, and wondered if it might possibly be linked to the mucus abnormality. A factor was found in the blood serum of some Cystic Fibrosis patients which, when added to the culture medium of oyster gill cells with cilia, resulted in disruption of the normal rhythmic beat of these minute hairs. This was the CDF (ciliary dyskinesia factor), one of the several 'CF factors' found in blood, saliva and various bodily secretions. A particular 'CF protein' or proteins were described, found not only in serum but in some cell secretions. This low molecular weight protein can be detected in Cystic Fibrosis patients and carriers, but it also occurs in some normal people, with considerable overlap, rendering it unsuitable for accurate testing. So, unfortunately, the 'basic defect' remained elusive.

The Cystic Fibrosis bronchial mucus also proved disappointing: it is certainly viscous but no more so than that found in other chronic lung infections unrelated to Cystic Fibrosis. Some disturbances in the movement of calcium in and out of various cells and body tissues were discovered, but again proved not to be the 'basic defect'. It seems that many of the biochemical findings were either normal variations or secondary effects of the disease.

Newborn Screening
During the period from 1964 to 1979, a number of research projects were mounted throughout the 'Cystic Fibrosis world' to explore possibilities for detecting Cystic Fibrosis soon after birth. This topic was dealt with briefly in Chapter Three. For some years there was doubt regarding the value of mass newborn screening and the accuracy of the techniques employed, and a general scepticism about cost effectiveness. Some tests gave as many as 15 to 20 per cent false negative results, which were all regarded as unacceptable; other tests gave varying numbers of false positive results, and the idea of mass screening fell into disrepute. There is now available a highly accurate blood spot test based on the pathology of the pancreas in Cystic Fibrosis, in which measurable amounts of the pancreatic digestive, trypsin,

leak into the blood. This test is simple, harmless and cost effective. Reports given at the Tenth International Congress in Sydney, in March 1988, indicate that infants diagnosed at birth by the updated test and kept under surveillance, with preventive treatment and improved nutritional care, have fared better than others not diagnosed until symptoms had become established.

It is now recognised that the lungs of Cystic Fibrosis people are normal at birth, so that diagnosis then could lead to better lung health, either by preventive treatment or by close monitoring of the infant for the earliest sign of any lung trouble, so that effective therapy may be applied at once.

Further prospective study projects are currently under way in Wales, the Midlands, Europe, Australia and Japan.

The 'Eighties
This epoch has seen tremendous advances in our understanding of Cystic Fibrosis, which have already resulted in active treatment becoming more effective and raising greater hopes for the future. The increased general public awareness of Cystic Fibrosis, with more extensive coverage in the media, has also helped in the overall support for Cystic Fibrosis people and their families.

The great scientific and medical advances have come in the following areas:

1 *Genetics.* The search for the 'CF gene' continues, conducted through by brilliant multinational co-operation.
2 *The Basic Defect.* Discovery of this will follow from identification of the gene and its products.
3 *Cell Transport.* Research in this field, combined with study of the nature of secretions, will lead to further understanding of the basic defect.
4 *Respiratory and Digestive Tracts.* Putting together the results of recent research, it is now becoming possible to compose a picture of how and why the pancreas, intestine, bile ducts and liver become disordered as they do; we are also beginning to form a coherent general impression of respiratory tract infection. This has posed

some unanswered questions for a long time—for example, 'Why pseudomonas, of all bacteria?' 'Why does the pseudomonas stick there all the time, in spite of the big guns of modern intensive antibiotic treatment?'

The year 1988 has been dubbed 'the year of the gene'. What has emerged from it? Apart from published reports in various scientific journals and reviews in *Cystic Fibrosis News*, the information that follows comes from scientific Cystic Fibrosis conferences, culminating in the Tenth International Cystic Fibrosis Congress in Sydney, Australia, in March 1988.

Genetics and Cell Epithelial Transport

Since 1980 the research into molecular biology, pioneered by Professor Bob Williamson and his group at St Mary's Hospital, Paddington, in co-operation with European, American and Canadian groups, has resulted in finding the 'Cystic Fibrosis gene' in Chromosome No 7, somewhere along its long arm. Already,this has enabled an accurate prenatal diagnosis to be made much earlier in pregnancy (at eight to ten weeks) than was previously possible, and has helped in the identification of Cystic Fibrosis carriers in at risk families. Further work should result in isolating the gene itself, with more accurate diagnostic tests in wider groups of people.

Cystic Fibrosis Carrier Mother and Carrier Father

The gene has been localised to No 7 Chromosome pair: each parent has one normal gene which is dominant over the Cystic Fibrosis gene, so that the gene product is made, and the parents are healthy. What is the 'gene product'? It is very likely to be a membrane protein, whose job is to regulate the passage of certain chemicals across the membranes of cells.

The theory of defective cell membrane transport of some essential body chemicals as being the 'basic defect' in Cystic Fibrosis has stimulated research in several centres. The Medical Research Council's unit at Cambridge, under Professor Eric Barnard, is using the egg cell of a toad to study the results of injecting human gene messengers. The behaviour of human genes involved in chemical transport can then be studied directly, comparing the results from normal genes with the effects of the Cystic Fibrosis gene.

Figure 8 shows what is known to happen in the sweat gland in Cystic Fibrosis. The sweat fluid comes from the blood circulating in the coil of the sweat gland, where chloride is present at a level of 100 units. As this fluid, which will emerge as sweat, travels up the sweat gland duct through the deeper layers of the skin, the membrane transport mechanism comes into action. The normal gene product coded from Chromosome No 7 effects the passage of chloride out from the duct into the surrounding tissues, and as the final sweat fluid emerges from the pore at outer skin level, the chloride content has fallen to 20 units. This mechanism is defective in Cystic Fibrosis, so that the surface sweat still contains 90–110 units of chloride; since sodium goes along with chloride in nature, the sweat is salty and this forms the basis of the Cystic Fibrosis diagnostic test. Some day, when the Cystic Fibrosis gene has been isolated, there will be a specific DNA diagnostic test available to back up and corroborate the sweat test.

Chloride is the most important membrane transfer chemical concerned; in the pancreas and lungs similar problems arise leading to thick, sticky and dehydrated secretions, perhaps involving other molecules such as calcium and bicarbonate.

So the combination of further genetic research plus detailed biochemical cell membrane investigations should lead reasonably soon to the discovery of the gene product and its normal function in regulating chloride transport. In Cystic Fibrosis, the abnormal gene at that particular part of Chromosome 7 produces either no protein at all, or else a defective product which does not do the job. Once this has been established, it will hopefully be possible to find a substitute to treat the Cystic Fibrosis patient, like Insulin for Diabetes, or Thyroxine for defective thyroid gland production.

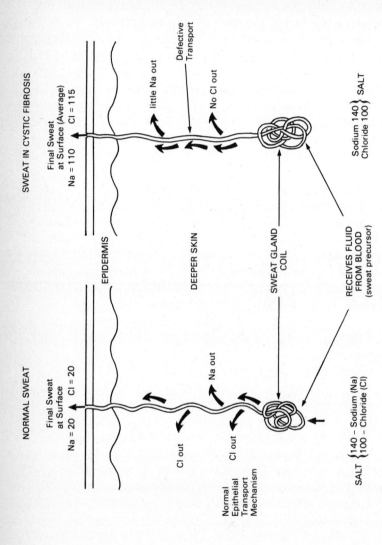

Figure 8. How the basic defect of cell membrane transport in Cystic Fibrosis shows in sweat.

The Movement Towards Self-Care

Now that more and more people with Cystic Fibrosis are attaining adulthood, there has been an understandable desire to shift the burden of treatment towards the individual in his home or place of study or work, so as to minimise time lost by attending hospital. I am all in favour of this culmination of the 'self-care advocacy' principle, but there are, or should be, some built-in safeguards. One is the need for regular contact with members of the Care Givers Network, whether this be a periodical check-up at the Cystic Fibrosis centre, talks with the medical social worker or clinical nurse specialist, and supervision of home intravenous or nebuliser equipment. The other necessity is supervision of physiotherapy and nutrition.

Guidelines for Respiratory Health

At the International Congress in Sydney, some guidelines were suggested for self-care. I am a fervent advocate of positive respiratory health, and admire the scientifically based modern respiratory physiotherapy which is both preventive and curative. A recommended schedule, to be carried out twice daily for 30 minutes, is as follows:

1   Breathing control, consisting of quiet, relaxed, deep breathing.
2   Chest expansion breathing exercises.
3   FET (forced expiratory technique): huffing and coughing. The 'huffing' should not be with a closed glottis, just making a lot of noise: the mouth should be open and the tongue slightly protruded, and the huffs should be timed to come not only as you begin to breathe out but towards the end of the exhalation, so as to get the most out of the smaller airways.
4   Always, after FET, comes breathing control—relaxed, as before.
5   Gravity-assisted postural drainage, combined with FET, has been shown to be a valuable combination technique.

The points made in these guidelines are taken from the keynote paper given by Barbara Webber of the Brompton Hospital, London, at the Sydney Conference.

Nutrition and Dietary Guidelines
The new thinking regarding nutrition and diet in Cystic Fibrosis was re-emphasised at Sydney. Malnutrition is still encountered, either generally or in specific nutrients such as protein, vitamins, trace elements and essential fatty acids. Positive attitudes are required towards variety in food intake, the value of milk in various forms, and the need for daily energy intake of 120–150 per cent of the usual recommended daily allowance.

A simple regime for adolescents and adults with Cystic Fibrosis was:

1 Eat a variety of foods each day.
2 Maintain a healthy body weight for your height and body build.
3 Eat FAT!
4 Eat sugar!
5 Use salt (you need it, obviously).
6 Enjoy milk in all its forms and recipes.
7 Minimal alcohol intake.
8 Maximum intake of cereals, milk, breads and protein foods.
9 Breastfeeding wherever possible for Cystic Fibrosis infants (see p. 50).

I would add to the above that you should not neglect dental care, and that you should take enough of the best pancreatic preparation (Creon, Pancrease) at intervals during meals to give you abdominal and digestive peace and comfort, you should also take Ranitidine if advised.

The following matters have also been raised recently:

1 The importance of the upper respiratory tract and its relationship to pulmonary infection.
2 The possible value of 'lingual lipase', a fat-digestive enzyme found in a gland beneath the tongue.

3 A new diagnostic test, measuring electrical potential difference across the nasal membranes. This is easily performed, painless and harmless, and the researchers at the Brompton Hospital say it is as accurate as the sweat test.

What Next?

For I dipt into the future, far as human eye can see,
Saw the Vision of the world, and all the wonder that
   would be.

So wrote Lord Tennyson in Queen Victoria's reign. I considered it a privilege to be invited to write this book and I trust I have fulfilled the duty that goes with privilege. My aim was to give parents, children, families, and now adolescent and adult people with Cystic Fibrosis, the basic facts that would enable them to achieve a fuller understanding of the condition. I have introduced the 'Shared-Care Network' which maintains a life-long commitment. I trust you can see what has been achieved and what we can all do about it together. Now, let me tell you what I believe will be achieved in the future.

As we approach the third millennium I foresee:

1 Genetic research will culminate in the isolation of the Cystic Fibrosis gene on Chromosome 7, leading to identification of the coded gene product, with the co-operation of:
2 Biochemical research on membrane transport, so that the missing or defective protein or enzyme—the basic defect—is uncovered, therefore:
3 A radical treatment analogous to Insulin or Thyroxine will become available to control the symptoms caused by the basic defect, so leading to a longer and better-quality life. At the same time:
4 Our treatment for lung infection, already greatly improved, will advance even further, thanks to the new genetic and biochemical knowledge, and to our deeper understanding of the apparent immunological upset in

the pseudomonas-infected lung. We have read about the heart/lung transplants: Some day, somehow, there will be a gene transplant.

12   THE TRUST

The Cystic Fibrosis Research Trust was born in 1964, the brain-child of the late John Panchaud, whose daughter had Cystic Fibrosis. Assisting at the birth of the Trust were two eminent consultants, Dr David Lawson and Dr Archie Norman, each of whom subsequently became Chairman of the Research and Medical Advisory Committee; both are now members of the Trust Council.

The Trust is Registered Charity No 281287. In the year following its founding, the infant organisation was highly honoured when Her Royal Highness Princess Alexandra, the Hon Mrs Angus Ogilvy, became Patron. Over the years since then, our Royal Patron has shown continued keen interest and understanding of all aspects of the Trust's work; for this, deep gratitude is expressed by all of us who have worked with the organisation.

The strategic objectives of the Trust have always been:

1   to finance research in order to find a complete cure for Cystic Fibrosis, and in the meantime to improve current methods of teatment;
2   to form regions, branches and groups throughout the United Kingdom for the purpose of helping and advising parents with the everyday problems of caring for Cystic Fibrosis children;
3   to educate the public about the disease and, through wider knowledge, to help promote earlier diagnosis.

Fund-raising is therefore a prime activity of the Trust. The regional branches and local groups have a reciprocal relationship with the Trust's headquarters in Kent, which provides them with constantly updated information on

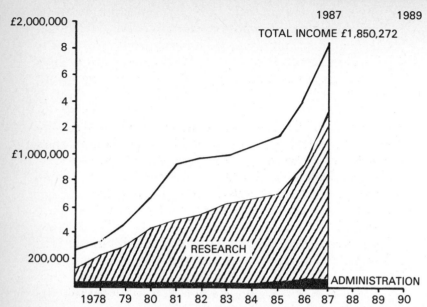

Figure 9. The Cystic Fibrosis Research Trust. Growth since 1977.

Cystic Fibrosis and gives practical help with organisation; in return they contribute their local effort and support for national fund-raising events. At present there are more than 86 groups and branches throughout the United Kingdom. There are also Regional Councils in Scotland, Northern Ireland and Wales. These groups, branches and regions provide three-quarters of the Trust's total income, which has increased from £750,000 in 1986–7 to £2,000,000 in 1987–8. A magnificent effort all round.

The Trust itself organises a number of sponsored events, and as you will see from Figure 9, the major part of its income has been devoted to the support of medical and scientific research.

The Research and Medical Advisory Committee comprises the Chairman and nine members, with varied professional expertise. This means clinical medicine, pathology, biochemistry, genetics and other scientific disciplines relevant to Cystic Fibrosis. A major part of the work of the RAMAC is to consider the applications for research grants and to recommend for financial support those judged to be of present or future value. In view of the broad strategic aims of uncovering the basic defect, this covers genetics, molecular biology and biochemistry, as well as ways of improving diagnostic methods, such as newborn screening, carrier detection and prenatal diagnosis. And, of course, all the time it is looking for improvements in our current clinical care of Cystic Fibrosis babies, school-children and the growing number of Cystic Fibrosis adolescents and adults.

It was my privilege to serve on the Committee for seven years under the chairmanship of the distinguished god-parents of the Trust, and with the help, advice and guid-ance of the Executive Director, Mr Ron Tucker, OBE, now retired, whose dedication to the cause, and tireless efforts, endeared him to parents, families and older patients as well as to all who served with him. He was also for many years Treasurer of the International Cystic Fibrosis (Mucoviscido-sis) Association, and was Co-ordinator of that highly suc-cessful International Cystic Fibrosis Congress at Brighton in 1984.

Some Research Projects Funded by the Trust
The Cystic Fibrosis gene has been much in the news lately, in scientific journals, the Press and the media. The work of Professor Bob Williamson and his group at St Mary's Hos-pital Medical School has been funded by the Trust, and this support is continuing, so that the gene localisation to the long arm of Chromosome 7 may be further defined and the gene protein product identified.

Two further projects are being funded. First, one with two eminent Cambridge scientists who are investigating how the Cystic Fibrosis gene produces its harmful effects and how the process could possibly be rectified or con-trolled. The second project is in the University College of Medicine, Cardiff, under the leadership of Dr Margaret McPherson. This group has already shown that the defect lies somewhere in the recipient cells of the body.

In the light of recent debates in the Commons, the problem of early prenatal diagnosis of Cystic Fibrosis leading to possible termination of pregnancy, already a subject of much discussion and research, is being further investigated by the chorionic villus biopsy technique described in Chapter 3. Funds for this have been allocated to genetic centres in Edinburgh, Cardiff, Manchester and London.

Funding for Cystic Fibrosis Clinical Fellowships is already established and further fellowship funding is being considered. There was a meeting of the Trust's Clinical Fellows in conjunction with the Hon Medical Advisers Conference at the Royal College of Physicians in September 1987, and all are agreed that this new field of activity is proving most successful. It ties in with the next area of funding—that of those centres of excellence known as regional (or possibly, in some cases, supra-regional) specialist Cystic Fibrosis centres. One of the first and best known of these is based at St James's University Hospital in Leeds (Europe's largest teaching hospital), headed by Dr Jim Littlewood. Recognition of this outstanding establishment has been shown by the recent award of an annual grant of £120,000 from the Yorkshire Regional Health Authority. The Trust has supported Dr Littlewood's scheme from the start and is hoping to encourage other regions to follow suit.

The Trust is also backing the work of Professor John Dodge and the British Paediatric Association, which advocated in their recent report, among other recommendations, the setting up of special Cystic Fibrosis 'Reference Centres'. Professor Dodge is compiling a computerised record of all Cystic Fibrosis patients in the United Kingdom, which will provide a database of great value to scientists and clinicians in the Cystic Fibrosis field, and therefore to the most important clients of the Trust—those with Cystic Fibrosis.

This work is being funded jointly by the Trust and the British Paediatric Association. Support is also being given, both moral and financial, to the recently introduced heart/

lung transplant operations for selected Cystic Fibrosis patients.

Welfare Activities

The Trust's Welfare Department provides both information and practical help to Cystic Fibrosis regional and branch organisations and to individual families who are uncertain about their benefits or are having difficulty with applications—for example, for Attendance Allowance.

The Caravan Holiday Fund is part of the practical help provided for Cystic Fibrosis families. Holiday camps with chalets and caravans are available in Hastings, South Wales, Fleetwood, Caister, Filey, Guiseley (Yorkshire) and Northern Ireland, with chalets in Lincoln and the Isle of Man.

Trust Meetings

Organising and hosting conferences forms an important and prestigious branch of the work of the Director and her staff. At the local level, lecture and discussion meetings are regularly held, well attended and generally much appreciated. Members of the Research and Medical Advisory Committee and other specialists will give an illustrated lecture on Cystic Fibrosis progress in general, or on some topic of current interest and importance. These visits are welcomed by the speakers, who have the opportunity to meet colleagues, parents and patients in parts of the United Kingdom away from their usual zone of operations. For 30–40 minutes after the talk, questions and answers are keenly appreciated by the audience. I am personally gratified to note the extent and depth of knowledge of Cystic Fibrosis which is exhibited by those attending, and I do not only mean professionals. Occasionally the meeting takes the form of about four shorter contributions by clinical and scientific workers, with a wide discussion on some topic of current interest, such as screening, prenatal diagnosis, management of respiratory infections, and so on.

At these regional meetings the Director is present, to confer with local officials, and is available for help and advice. After the medical scientific part is over, she gives an update on Cystic Fibrosis matters, including the results of the recent functions and notice of future fund-raising events.

Trust Publications
A series of booklets is currently available, published by the Trust and written by health professionals for parents of Cystic Fibrosis children, their families and the children themselves. The authors are chosen for their special knowledge and experience in various aspects of Cystic Fibrosis, and the series covers all stages in the treatment and management of the disease.

Cystic Fibrosis. This booklet tells the whole story from day one, and is the mainstay leaflet to help new parents.

Genetics and Tests During Pregnancy. This explains the genetic inheritance of Cystic Fibrosis, prenatal diagnosis procedures currently available, and the methods of carrier detection which are being investigated.

Cystic Fibrosis and You. A very popular booklet for children with Cystic Fibrosis—but of interest also to families, schoolteachers and many others.

Know the Facts. A recently updated, small four-fold leaflet which answers all the basic questions.

The Physical Treatment of Cystic Fibrosis. An illustrated booklet giving full details of up-to-date methods of physiotherapy. Written by two of the country's leading physiotherapists.

Nutritional Management of Cystic Fibrosis. Full details of nutrition and diet with delicious and appetising recipes.

Nutrition for the Adult with Cystic Fibrosis. An adult version of the Nutritional leaflet described above.

Immunisation and Infectious Diseases. Advice on immunisation at all ages.

Cystic Fibrosis and the Use of Jet Nebulisers. This booklet gives a detailed description of how to use jet nebulisers, and how to look after them.

Fertility, Pregnancy and Contraception in Cystic Fibrosis. A well-informed and frank discussion of many of the problems facing the young Cystic Fibrosis adult.

How Social Workers Can Help the Family. Written by a social worker from the Brompton Hospital, this is a valuable reminder of how helpful social workers can be.

Guide to Government and Voluntary Help. A guide through some of the complexities of the DSS, and help with other problems. There is a tear-off page for Cystic Fibrosis job applicants to hand to potential employers if they wish.

Attendance Allowance. A full explanation of this allowance and how you should claim for it.

Cystic Fibrosis and School. A useful guide with sections addressed to the schoolteachers.

Growing Up with Cystic Fibrosis. A guide for the young adult, soon to be supplemented by a series of new leaflets currently being produced by the Association of Cystic Fibrosis Adults.

In addition to these booklets for families and patients, the Trust publishes *Cystic Fibrosis News*, a magazine for all readers, issued six times a year; and *Cystic Fibrosis Now*, an occasional newspaper full of news and articles on special topics.

For professionals there are books on proceedings of international conferences, short films on loan, and a tape-slide programme intended for students but of interest also for all health care professionals. The tape-slide review was produced in the Department of Medical Illustration, University Hospital of Wales, Cardiff.

The Trust organises and funds regular meetings and conferences of scientific research workers and the biennial conference of regional and district Honorary Medical Advisers.

Association of Cystic Fibrosis Adults (UK)

The ACFA(UK) was formed in 1983. The aims and objectives of this association are:

1 To help the Cystic Fibrosis adult lead as full and independent a life as possible.
2 To promote the exchange of information.
3 To act as a forum for improving the management of problems encountered by Cystic Fibrosis adults, both medical and otherwise.
4 To provide encouragement for all those with Cystic Fibrosis and their families.
5 To assist wherever possible the efforts of the Cystic Fibrosis Research Trust.

The Trust has supported ACFA from the start, and now helps in the production of the regular and popular newsletter, preparation of their own leaflets and various other activities. The newsletter, produced quarterly, consists of a medical article, general information and details of events and meetings. There is also a correspondence column.

The ACFA steering Committee was dissolved in August 1987, and a new Management Committee was formed. The main appointments were as follows: Chairman, Treasurer, Secretary and Chief Editor, Medical Liaison Officer, '89 Conference Organiser, Executive Committee and International Representative, Welfare Officer, Publicity Officer. The non-voting, non-Cystic Fibrosis positions were: Honorary Medical Adviser, Cystic Fibrosis Research Trust Representative, and Administration Officer (based at the Cystic Fibrosis Research Trust headquarters in Kent).

The first national conference of ACFA was held in Mansfield College, Oxford, in April 1987, and the following autumn delegates attended the international meeting held during the European Working Group's annual meeting in Hungary.

The increasing and widespread interest in Cystic Fibrosis was exemplified by that gathering in Budapest. Hosted by the Hungarian Paediatric Society and its Cystic Fibrosis group, the various sessions comprised the 14th Annual Meeting of the European Working Group for Cystic Fibrosis, the 21st Annual Meeting of the International Cystic Fibrosis (Mucoviscidosis) Association and the Third Conference of the International Association of Cystic Fibrosis Adults.

All these multinational Cystic Fibrosis institutions are supported in various ways by the Cystic Fibrosis Research Trust. The International Cystic Fibrosis Association was set up in 1964, following the initiative of the Canadian and American Cystic Fibrosis Foundations. The Fifth International Congress was held in Cambridge in 1969 and the Ninth in Brighton in 1984, the Chairman of the medical programme committee being Dr David Lawson, and the whole event hosted by the UK Trust.

At present there are some forty countries whose Cystic Fibrosis organisations are members or associate members of the ICF(M)A. The international aims include the interchange of ideas and information on research into the basic cause of Cystic Fibrosis, its possible prevention or control, and eventual cure. Meetings of the various Cystic Fibrosis groups, Government bodies and World Health Organisation representatives help to promote knowledge of the prevalence of Cystic Fibrosis, and help in national plans for the medical care and welfare support for all patients and their families.

Cystic Fibrosis is becoming more widely known and better understood, raising our hopes for the future. I earnestly advise all Cystic Fibrosis families—parents, children, adolescents and adult patients—to support the Trust and join their local group.

The Trust 'Team'
Patron: HRH Princess Alexandra, the Hon Mrs Angus Ogilvy
Hon Life Presidents: The Rt Hon Lord Cook, KStJ, JP, Joseph Levy, CBE, BEM.
COUNCIL
President: Sir John Batten, KCVO, MD, FRCP

It is in a large part due to the personality, total dedication to the job and general empathy of the Director and her staff that the Cystic Fibrosis Research Trust has been 'Highly Commended' by the charities world, in due recognition of the enormous amount of work it does to improve the outlook for Cystic Fibrosis sufferers and their families.

GLOSSARY

AMNIOTIC FLUID	The fluid surrounding the baby in the womb.
ARTHROPATHY	See HPOA (Hypertrophic Pulmonary Osteoarthropathy).
AUTOSOME	Body cells—all chromosomes other than the sex chromosomes.
CHORIONIC VILLI	The rumpled outer surface of the membranes surrounding the baby in the womb. Part of the chorion forms the placenta later in pregnancy.
CILIARY DYSKINESIS FACTOR	A substance able to disrupt the synchronised movement of the cilia (the airways are lined with minute hairs which move rhythmically to clear secretions).
CYTOPLASM	The fluid substance inside a cell.
DNA	(Deoxyribonucleic acid.) The major component of genetic material. The biological molecule that codes for all the information needed to construct a human being from a single fertilised egg.
DIOS	(Distal Intestinal Obstruction Syndrome.) There is no connection between the cause of DIOS and Meconium Ileus Equivalent.
EMPHYSEMA	Permanent overdistention of the alveolae in the lungs.
EMPYEMA	A condition in which pus forms in the pleural cavity—the space between the chest wall and the lung.
GENE	A specifically coded length of DNA.
HETEROZYGOTES	The carriers of the abnormal gene, who do not have Cystic Fibrosis themselves.
HOMOZYGOTES	Those who have inherited the Cystic Fibrosis gene from both parents, and as a result have Cystic Fibrosis.

HPOA	(Hypertrophic Pulmonary Osteoarthropathy.) Pain in the large joints.
INTUSSUSCEPTION	A common variety is called ileo-colic, and occurs when a section of the small intestine folds into the adjoining large gut leading downstream to the bowel, endangering its blood supply.
MECONIUM ILEUS	An obstruction of the small intestine at birth. Meconium is a sticky, dry substance which blocks up the bowel passage.
MECONIUM ILEUS EQUIVALENT	Intestinal obstruction.
MCT	(Medium chain triglycerides.) A consumable oil which can be absorbed directly into the bloodstream from the intestine.
MUCOLYTIC	Substance capable of thinning mucus. It may do this by increasing the water content of the mucus or by breaking the chemical bonds between sulphur and hydrogen.
MUCOVISCIDOSIS	Another name for Cystic Fibrosis.
NUCLEUS	The control centre of a cell.
PANCREAS	Lies behind the stomach and provides the digestive juices through the pancreatic ducts.
PERISTALSIS	The 'muscular wave' which causes matter to move along the intestines.
PROLAPSED RECTUM	Sometimes occurs in infants with Cystic Fibrosis. Malabsorption of fat with frequent stools causes the inner lining of the rectum to protrude through the anus.
RECESSIVE ·	The description of a gene the effects of which are masked by the presence of the dominant counterpart in the same cell.
THE SWEAT TEST	A painless test carried out on sweat obtained from the skin surface to measure the sodium chloride content. An aid to the diagnosis of Cystic Fibrosis.
VISCOUS	Sticky.

BIBLIOGRAPHY

BATTEN, J., HODSON, M., and NORMAN, A. P. *Cystic Fibrosis*, Baillière Tindall, 1983.

BURTON, L. *The Family Life of a Sick Child*, Routledge & Kegan Paul, 1975. Paperback.

CAPEWELL, G. *Cystic Fibrosis*, Office of Health Economics, 1986. Paperback with diagrams.

DODGE, J., and GOODCHILD, M. (eds). *Cystic Fibrosis: Manual of Diagnosis and Management*, Baillière Tindall, 1985. Second edition, paperback.

HARRIS, A., and SUPER, M. (eds). *Cystic Fibrosis: The Facts*, Oxford University Press, 1987. With diagrams.

LAWSON, D. (ed). *Cystic Fibrosis: Horizons*, Proceedings of the Ninth International Cystic Fibrosis Congress, Brighton, England, John Wiley & Sons, 1984.

PETTENUZZO, B. *I Have Cystic Fibrosis*, Franklin Watts, 1988. Written with Victoria Haines, aged 12.

THOMAS, S. *Genetic Risk*, Penguin Books, 1986. Paperback.

'Current Clinical Management of Cystic Fibrosis', in *Journal of the Royal Society of Medicine*, No. 12, 1986.

Recent Advances in Management of Cystic Fibrosis. Symposium held by the Section of Paediatrics of the Royal Society of Medicine. Royal Society of Medicine, 1987. Paperback.

INDEX